'Barbara Pizer's book is riveting. Her detailed use of self is evocative and enriching. Her thinking, anchored in Body Words, is novel, deep, and compelling. She achieves an extraordinary depth of perspective in theory and practice, demonstrating an incredible ability to immerse herself in clinical challenges, to conceptualize them, and meet them. It's a must-read for all clinicians.'

Hazel Ipp, PhD, *chief editor emeritus,*
Psychoanalytic Dialogues; *vice president, IARPP*

'Open this book and enter a world of experience. As one of the masters of the practice and theory of Relational Psychoanalysis, Barbara Pizer conveys in exquisite detail how psychoanalysis moves and changes people's lives. She practices and teaches the art of engagement, where feeling and expression, whether verbal or not, are the embodied center of clinical work. You will feel immersed in the living moment of analytic work. More important, you will learn how the shared knots of repetition loosen and transform into a more open way of engaging and living creatively as well.'

Jack Foehl, PhD, *joint editor-in-chief,* Psychoanalytic Dialogues;
president, Boston Psychoanalytic Society and Institute

'Pizer's book demonstrates her astute capacity to put the world of the patient-therapist relationship before us. Her innovative ideas for how to engage successfully in the dyad are perfect for both experienced and new clinicians. Body Words is an accurate, evocative expression of mind-brain-body connection crucial for a contemporary emphasis on nonlinear process and systems thinking. Finally, there is the poetry in Pizer's prose that her old readers have come to expect and new readers, dreading theory-heavy, unimaginative writing, will welcome.'

Estelle Shane, PhD, *training and supervising analyst*
and faculty member, Insitute of Contemporary Psychoanalysis,
Los Angeles, and the New Center for Psychoanalysis, Los Angeles

T0383650

Body Words and the Analyst's Use of Self

In this book, it becomes impossible to stand apart from the analytic field as abstract concepts, such as dissociation, intersubjectivity, and unconscious communication, as well as newly coined ones, like "Relational (K)not" and "Body Words," come alive through a vivid unfolding of analytic process.

You are invited into the mind of the analyst as she draws from reverie, memory, and affect to inspire offerings that enliven the moment, moving the analytic pair forward in affective freedom and self-definition. Body Words identify the subjective linkages we make to describe *experiencing* within and between self and other that lead us to know whether we or our patient are delivering the message in a manner that feels real. Each chapter illustrates how Pizer arrived at this important concept and others in a way that is full of rich, experience-near clinical moments that posed significant challenges.

Body Words and the Analyst's Use of Self is a rare window that allows readers—new and seasoned clinicians of various theoretical persuasions— to become intimate witnesses to the analyst's subjectivity and the creativity of the analytic partnership.

Barbara Pizer, EdD, ABPP, is faculty, personal and supervising analyst, and former board member of the Massachusetts Institute for Psychoanalysis; assistant clinical professor of Psychology, Department of Psychiatry, Harvard Medical School; associate editor of *Psychoanalytic Dialogues*; and in private practice in Cambridge, Massachusetts.

Psychoanalysis in A New Key Book Series
Donnel Stern
Series Editor

When music is played in a new key, the melody does not change, but the notes that make up the composition do: change in the context of continuity, continuity that perseveres through change. Psychoanalysis in a New Key publishes books that share the aims psychoanalysts have always had, but that approach them differently. The books in the series are not expected to advance any particular theoretical agenda, although to this date most have been written by analysts from the interpersonal and relational orientations.

The most important contribution of a psychoanalytic book is the communication of something that nudges the reader's grasp of clinical theory and practice in an unexpected direction. Psychoanalysis in a New Key creates a deliberate focus on innovative and unsettling clinical thinking. Because that kind of thinking is encouraged by exploration of the sometimes surprising contributions to psychoanalysis of ideas and findings from other fields, Psychoanalysis in a New Key particularly encourages interdisciplinary studies. Books in the series have married psychoanalysis with dissociation, trauma theory, sociology, and criminology. The series is open to the consideration of studies examining the relationship between psychoanalysis and any other field—for instance, biology, literary and art criticism, philosophy, systems theory, anthropology, and political theory.

But innovation also takes place within the boundaries of psychoanalysis, and Psychoanalysis in a New Key therefore also presents work that reformulates thought and practice without leaving the precincts of the field. Books in the series focus, for example, on the significance of personal values in psychoanalytic practice, on the complex interrelationship between the analyst's clinical work and personal life, on the consequences for the clinical situation when patient and analyst are from different cultures, and on the need for psychoanalysts to accept the degree to which they knowingly satisfy their own wishes during treatment hours, often to the patient's detriment.

A full list of all titles in this series is available at:

https://www.routledge.com/Psychoanalysis-in-a-New-Key-Book-Series/book-series/LEAPNKBS

Body Words and the Analyst's Use of Self

Transforming the Unspeakable in Clinical Process

Barbara Pizer

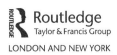

Routledge
Taylor & Francis Group

LONDON AND NEW YORK

Cover Art: Helene Schjerfbeck, *The Red-Haired Girl II*, 1915. Owner, Gösta Serlachius Fine Arts Foundation, Mänttä, Finland.

Photo, Jussi Tiainen, 2016.

First published 2024
by Routledge
4 Park Square, Milton Park, Abingdon, Oxon OX14 4RN

and by Routledge
605 Third Avenue, New York, NY 10158

Routledge is an imprint of the Taylor & Francis Group, an informa business

British Library Cataloguing-in-Publication Data
A catalogue record for this book is available from the British Library

Library of Congress Cataloging-in-Publication Data
Names: Pizer, Barbara, author.
Title: Body words and the analyst's use of self: transforming the unspeakable in clinical process / Barbara Pizer.
Description: Abingdon, Oxon; New York, NY: Routledge, 2024. | Series: Psychoanalysis in a new key | Includes bibliographical references and index. |
Identifiers: LCCN 2023047781 (print) | LCCN 2023047782 (ebook) | ISBN 9781032666297 (hardback) | ISBN 9781032666280 (paperback) | ISBN 9781032666303 (ebook)
Subjects: LCSH: Psychoanalysis. | Psychotherapist and patient.
Classification: LCC RC506 .P569 2024 (print) | LCC RC506 (ebook) | DDC 616.89/17--dc23/eng/20240119
LC record available at https://lccn.loc.gov/2023047781
LC ebook record available at https://lccn.loc.gov/2023047782

ISBN: 9781032666297 (hbk)
ISBN: 9781032666280 (pbk)
ISBN: 9781032666303 (ebk)

DOI: 10.4324/9781032666303

Typeset in Times New Roman
by Deanta Global Publishing Services, Chennai, India

For my husband, Stuart,
who taught me to value my thoughts
and has always helped me to find the words,

and for my children,
Andrea, David, and Maya,
with gratitude for their loving support

Contents

Acknowledgments

Donnel B. Stern, whose own writings have inspired me for more than three decades, has been a patient, persistent, and loving friend to me and to this book. For a decade, perhaps more, he has affirmed me, nudged me, prompted me gently to finally complete this book. Donnel's belief in my work has sustained me through years of doubt, shyness, and resistance. I am immensely grateful.

Stuart Pizer, my husband and partner in creativity, contributed profoundly to the evolution of my writing through our coteaching, our daily dialogues, and his own writing. Always respectful of the origin of ideas within me, Stuart has been intrinsic to the unfolding of these chapters.

Suzi Naiburg has been essential to the realization of this book. I am the fortunate beneficiary of her tenacious and loving encouragement. Widely recognized as an expert on psychoanalytic writing, author of an important book on particular forms of psychoanalytic writing, and coach to many a published author, Suzi has been a devoted support in tasks ranging from careful textual editing to the minutiae of manuscript preparation that were, frankly, beyond me. Thank you, Suzi, for making this happen.

In particular, individual ways, I am grateful for the contributions of Hazel Ipp, Ilse Tebbetts, Fern Massar, Andrea Massar, Jack Foehl, Estelle Shane, and my first mentor, the late George Goethals. I wish Paul Russell were alive today to thank him personally. As instructor, supervisor, and inspiring author, Paul rendered seminal ideas that were always so close to essential clinical reality.

And at Routledge, Georgina Clutterbuck has been a model of gracious hospitality, patience, and kind flexibility. In correspondence, I always felt that a lovely person sat at the other end of the e-mail.

Finally, I am grateful to Joel Ruimy for the intellect, skill, and care he brought to creating an extraordinary index.

Copyright Acknowledgments

Chapter 6. "'Eva, Get the Goldfish Bowl': Affect and Intuition in the Analytic Relationship" by Barbara Pizer (2023). *Psychoanalytic Dialogues*, *33*(5): 603–618. Reprinted by permission of the publisher (Taylor & Francis, Ltd. http://www.tandfonline.com).

Chapter 7. "From Black Hole to Potential Space: Discussion of Barbara Pizer's 'Eva, Get the Goldfish Bowl': Affect and Intuition in the Analytic Relationship" by Stuart Pizer (2023). *Psychoanalytic Dialogues*, *33*(5):619–625. Reprinted by permission of the publisher (Taylor & Francis, Ltd. http://www.tandfonline.com).

Chapter 8. "Risk and Potential in Analytic Disclosure: Can the Analyst Make 'The Wrong Thing' Right?" by Barbara Pizer (2006). *Contemporary Psychoanalysis*, *42*(1), 31–40. Reprinted by permission of the publisher (Taylor & Francis, Ltd. http://www.tandfonline.com).

Chapter 9. "The Heart of the Matter in Matters of the Heart: Power and Intimacy in Analytic and Couples Relationships" by Barbara Pizer (2008). *International Journal of Psychoanalytic Self Psychology*, *3*(3), 304–319. Reprinted by permission of the publisher (Taylor & Francis, Ltd. http://www.tandfonline.com).

Chapter 10. "A Clinical Exploration of Moving Anger Forward: Intimacy, Anger, and Creative Freedom" by Barbara Pizer (2014). *Psychoanalytic Dialogues*, *24*(1), 14–28. Reprinted by permission of the publisher (Taylor & Francis, Ltd. http://www.tandfonline.com).

Chapter 13. "'Why Can't We Be Lovers?' When the Price of Love Is Loss of Love: Boundary Violations in Clinical Context" by Barbara Pizer (2017). *Psychoanalytic Psychology*, *34*(2), 163–168. Reprinted by permission of the publisher (American Psychological Association. www.apa.org/pubs/journal/pap); permission conveyed through Copyright Clearance Center, Inc.

Chapter 14. "Not Me: The Vicissitudes of Aging" by Barbara Pizer (2019). *Psychoanalytic Dialogues*, *29*(5), 536–542. Reprinted by permission of the publisher (Taylor & Francis, Ltd. http://www.tandfonline.com).

Chapter 15. "Writing, Repetition, and Body Words: Transformation in Clinical Process" by Barbara Pizer (2021). *Psychoanalysis, Self, and Context*, *16*(2), 154–162. Reprinted by permission of the publisher (Taylor & Francis, Ltd. http://www.tandfonline.com).

Foreword

Donnel B. Stern

I suppose it's always justified to argue that whomever you're reading really doesn't write like anyone else. But in Barbara Pizer's case, it's more true than usual. Nobody, *nobody* writes like Barbara. There are writers of fiction who write *more* like Barbara than any psychoanalyst does. But nobody in psychoanalysis writes like Barbara. And because Barbara's themes are psychoanalytic, it really isn't true to say, as I just did, that there are fiction writers who write *more* like Barbara than any psychoanalyst. Fiction writers have it easy in the same way traditional psychoanalytic writers do: their form has long been associated with a particular range of styles. In fiction, of course, that range is very wide. Style is always part of content, so that writers are entirely free to make their means of presentation a contribution to the effect on the reader. In psychoanalysis, on the other hand, because most writing is intended to be instrumental, just a way to convey content, most articles and books are written in a narrow, academic style that tends to be desiccated and uninteresting. That writing is no more than a means to an end. There are important exceptions to this rule, and the exceptions have proliferated in recent decades. Among well-known psychoanalytic writers, one thinks of Winnicott, Bion (who is expressive, even if sometimes turgid), Ogden, McLaughlin, and too many others to name. But they remain the exceptions and not the rule. And they must therefore buck the trend. In order to tell things their way, they must insist, and not infrequently they face(d) resistance.

Barbara has faced her share of resistance too, but she has persevered, offering us between these covers real riches—clinical riches, yes, absolutely, and I will have more to say about them, but also riches having to do with the pleasure of reading. The book you hold in your hands is a deeply serious endeavor that certainly does need to be studied for its clinical lessons, but it is also well suited, if you are the right kind of person, to entertain you in a comfortable chair on a rainy afternoon, or on a day at the beach when you want something more substantial than a bestseller but just can't face, for the moment, the scientistic tone of so much psychoanalytic writing.

Now, before I can say anything more about the style of the writing here, I must say something about the book's content. The psychoanalytic papers that make up the book were written over the last thirty years, and so we can say that, up to this point, these chapters are (in tandem with her clinical work and teaching, of course) Barbara's life work. You will see as you read them that while each chapter has very specific and explicit roots in what Barbara was doing clinically at the time it was written, together they manifest an abiding set of clinical interests. The best and simplest ways to refer to these themes are provided by Barbara herself in her title. First, take "the analyst's use of self." These essays all address how the analyst uses her own experience—always her experience *with the patient*, but very often memories and new formulations of her own life that her experience with the patient provokes her to create or revisit. And then consider the other phrase in her title, "transforming the unspeakable in clinical process." The analyst's self, in other words, somehow must be used by the psychoanalyst in such a way that the difficulties that brought the patient to treatment, and that cannot be known, inhabited, or fully felt, can become living, breathing parts of the patient's life—using "Body Words," in the phrase Barbara introduces in Chapter 15. These themes—using the self and transforming the unspeakable—lead Barbara to examine other topics too, but always within this larger context. We learn Barbara's perspective on a variety of issues: the analyst's self-disclosure, liveliness and deadness in analytic relatedness, enactment (Barbara leans here, and elsewhere, on the work of her mentor Paul Russell, who referred to enactment, usefully and colorfully, as "the crunch"), the roles of power and intimacy in analytic relatedness, trauma and dissociation, boundary violations in psychoanalysis, and aging.

One theme that is never far from Barbara's consideration is the vitality of the analytic relationship—its quality of aliveness or deadness. In Chapter 3, for example, we find Barbara differentiating mutual detachment in analytic relatedness—what she calls "(k)nots," condensing in this pun Laing's "knots" with a different kind of (knot that is the absence of emotional connection, a not—from the more dramatic enactments that deserve to be called "crunches." In Chapter 11, we find Barbara helping Aaren (yes, with an e—and that will be explained when you read the chapter) to stay emotionally alive. And so on, in one chapter after another, each chapter contributing to the development of the theme.

I said that I needed to give you some idea of this book's content before I could say anything more about its style. In alerting you to Barbara's fascination with affective aliveness, and to the centrality of the idea in these essays, I have now said what I needed to say in order to convey exactly what to me is *really* special about what Barbara does on the page: it is her writing of clinical material, her presentation of her work with her patients.

Barbara's clinical writing is good in the way that good fiction is good. It is alive, specific, and particular. The details pop. And many of those details that pop are emotional details. Anyone who writes can tell you that conveying the affective life of your characters, without just clunkily saying what they are feeling, is the art and craft of writing. Barbara does this superbly. When she writes about what she feels in a session, or what she imagines the patient feels, you are given a real sense of what that is like. In "'Eva, Get the Goldfish Bowl'" (Chapter 6), the conversation between Barbara and Julian, her patient, is a marvel of phenomenological inquiry. We read a bit of what Julian said, and then Barbara tells us what she was thinking in that moment; and then Julian speaks again, and again Barbara fills us in about her own state of mind. This goes on long enough to give us a ringside seat at the session. Or something more intimate than that, actually, because a ringside seat wouldn't allow us to appreciate Barbara's internal experience. A colleague of Barbara's said that these pages are innovative enough that they establish a new form of clinical writing. She may be right. They are, at the very least, a profound pleasure to read, and an example of what language can do in the right hands. And all of this, mind you, happens within the larger context of the essay, which is this:

> Beyond our own analysis, our patients may awaken in us long-dormant memories of shame and pain and joy, experiences that serve—for a brief time—to cut through loneliness, experiences that may well vitalize, enrich, and enliven who we are, who we've come to be.

Beautifully expressed. I quote it not only because of that, though, but also because I want to leave you with the impression that, however marvelous Barbara's clinical writing may be, it always serves a larger purpose. And that, to my mind, makes it all the more moving.

Let me cite one more example of Barbara's characterizations. I could choose many. I alight on the beautiful evocation of the relationship between Barbara and her patient Doreen in Chapter 15, "Body Words: Transforming the Unspeakable in Clinical Process." I quote a brief passage:

> I am shocked to discover myself unable to conjure Doreen's face. And yet I have a sense of certain modes of being that her face gets into, like eyebrows slightly raised, eyelids half-mast along with a certain sideways glance that marks disdain; or her closed-mouth, tight-lipped so-called smile that tells me *she has had enough of that!*

Wow. *That* is a particular person, isn't it? And "certain modes of being that her face gets into"! Perfect.

Barbara coins the term "Body Words" in this same chapter:

> Body Words gather up the fragments of what may be only vaguely felt at first, emerging into a word, gesture, or phrase that suddenly appears from nowhere, "unbidden" (Stern, 1997). Body Words signal a transformative experience heading toward increased integration of inner and outer processes, of direct experience and representation.

Body Words anchor one pole of a dialectic: they grow from the body and are therefore unmistakably vital, alive, and authentic. The other pole of the dialectic Barbara calls "repetition compulsion," after her mentor Paul Russell, who taught that this phenomenon is the opposite of "relationship," and that relationship is the aim of every psychoanalytic treatment—an authentic, affectively alive experience of oneself and the other. Russell also taught that forward movement from repetition compulsion to relationship can be prevented by the analyst's resistance to what the patient is feeling. Much of Barbara's clinical presentations are explorations of her own resistance to the patient's feeling.

In this "Body Words" chapter, written very recently and therefore heir to all of Barbara's thoughts over the last decades, all three of the themes I have tried to cover in these few words of introduction are present—the analyst's use of self, transforming the unspeakable, and vitality and aliveness. I suspect that readers are reminded of Winnicott, the grandparent of psychoanalytic interest in vitality. For Winnicott, vitality and authenticity had everything to do with the body. He referred to the "psyche/soma," and argued that "mind" is a desiccated thing, detached from the body. Because of certain early states of relatedness with caretakers, "mind" cannot give expression to "true self" in the way that, because of the preservation of its origins in the body, is sometimes possible for "psyche."

Barbara's work is very much in this Winnicottian tradition. But Barbara has added something. For Winnicott, the analyst offers what he called "environmental provision," essential for the eventual experience of vitality in the experience of people whose early relationships have been traumatic. But environmental provision, despite being a responsive acceptance, is not a whole relationship with another adult, with all the feelings that a whole relationship must contain. Furthermore, the outcome of environmental provision, while it is mediated by the analytic relationship, is understood to take place in the patient's psyche.

But for Barbara environmental provision would be an incomplete description of what the analyst must offer the patient. Barbara is expounding in this book a more thoroughly relational view, in which treatment is a project of "reclamation and growth of the availability of Body Words in *both* participants" (emphasis added). Each participant needs to find and respect the full range of affective reactions human beings can have to one another. Psychoanalytic treatment for Barbara is best described as the transformation of the analytic process between the two participants from repetition compulsion to relationship.

Chapter 1

Introduction

Body Words and the Analyst's Use of Self: Transforming the Unspeakable in Clinical Process is the outcome of ongoing efforts to set down in writing what I believe are the necessary qualities that permit me to engage another in the work and play of growth and healing. The concept of Body Words is central to this process, my book, and my life's work—over fifty years as a psychologist and psychoanalyst, supervisor, teacher, and mentor. These pages reflect my emergent understanding of clinical process from the perspective of an evolving Relational Psychoanalysis.

As I articulate in Chapter 15, I use the term *Body Words* to identify the subjective linkages we make to describe *experiencing*. Developmentally, Body Words evolve from the first conversations held within each one of us as we attempt to make meaning of the world as it enters through our senses from the outside and as we answer to it with feelings from the inside. It is a conversation that develops naturally enough until or unless something interrupts, like trauma or exposure to shame. Or maybe an early pattern of misrecognition begins to skew the internal dialogue, or subtle punishments inhibit. Any and all of these strictures have an impact on the words or gestures that we make or experience, gradually, imperceptibly, cutting us loose from what once was truly felt, encouraging forgetfulness of how or what we meant to say—if anything at all. The end result becomes a disembodied language either so shocking or by now so ordinary that we dissociatively disattend the unhooked dialogue in others and ourselves until or unless we are lucky enough to stumble on a particular moment when we are jolted awake or aware.

Body Words is my particular metaphorical term for the experience within and between self and other that leads us to know whether we or the person talking to us is delivering his message in a manner that feels real,

DOI: 10.4324/9781032666303-1

or more generally, if the contact we pick up between ourselves and others has a genuine ring to it. By assigning an interactive double name to the phenomenon, I hope to heighten awareness of a dual process involving both the body and the mind without privileging one over the other. Body Words is the corporate version, the communication aspect, the relational edge of the mind/body/brain.

Body is meant to signify the internal corporeal location wherein genuine affective experiences arise and are discretely felt but remain evanescent until or unless words grab hold. *Words*, in this context, serve as a metaphor for affective communication—both verbal and nonverbal—within and between bodies, linking the internal and external worlds. The metaphor bridges affect and cognition. While heartfelt sensations occur in the body, words—a delineating form of expressiveness—provide the containers that permit one's affects to travel around and out.

Body Words gather up the fragments of what may be only vaguely felt at first, emerging into a word, gesture, or phrase that suddenly appears from nowhere, "unbidden" (Stern, 1997). Body Words signal a transformative experience heading toward increased integration of inner and outer processes, of direct experience and representation. What I call Body Words is an experience I think of as having the shape of an arc. I use Body Words to indicate the peak of an experience that travels from inside to outside.

The circle or process arc of a Body Words experience, in which a body sense is linked to word representation (symbolization, formulation) that becomes communicable to self or other, is always moving. First, a slight interruption of ordinary being makes a bid for attention, a kind of inkling, an itch, a tension in the body that may be ignored, denied, dissociated, or distanced by isolation of affect. But if we choose to turn our attention to that embodied inkling (Gendlin, 1962, 1978, would call it "felt referent"), we become open to discover or have the potential to find words that emerge in our minds—Body Words. This part of the process would be called "carrying forward" in Gendlin's (1978) model of focusing, or in Donnel B. Stern's (1997) terms "formulating experience." Body Words (gesture or language expressing bodily feelings) can be received and responded to (by analyst or self), and a close observing or listening to the words may induce a further embodied response (for Gendlin, 1978, "referent movement"). Thus, the circle of Body Words experience may continue as an emergent process that Russell (1996) would call "affective connectedness."

The Analyst's Use of Self

In my own journey from body intensities to word clarity, at about age six or seven I seem to have adopted an interim measure. My semiblindness from over oxygenation in the incubator was not recognized or diagnosed until I was eight or nine. I was simply the girl who got arithmetic, reading, or class participation all jumbled. With a reputation in my family as "over-emotional," I was pervasively exposed to shame. Often when words would not come, I wept.

Then I discovered that I could express myself by playing a recording of "Peter and the Wolf" and embodying the narrative by dancing each of the characters. My body in movement would depict all the emotions that the characters represented. Now it was *Peter's* carefree spirit of rebellion and adventure that got conveyed—not mine; *Peter* who *freed* himself from his grandfather's cautious restrictions! And soon the twittery observer bird would appear on the scene, would fly down and start an argument with the impetuous duck, who jumps out of the pond only to be swallowed up whole by the greedy wolf! (So much for making protest!) And then the stalwart hunters come gunning out of the woods to capture the wolf that Peter had already roped by its tail. Major humiliation here!

As a child, my vocabulary was the language of the body. Music and movement came naturally. Expressing myself verbally did not. So it is a thrill for me that at this stage of my life I can share with you my accumulated clinical and conceptual understanding in words. Body Words.

The chapters that follow trace the evolution of my thinking, beginning in an earlier era of the development of Relational Psychoanalysis. Hence, some of the concepts that I introduced that were risky or revolutionary at the time are now accepted and even part of the mainstream, e.g., making the analyst's illness speakable, including the personal in our professional writing. Reveries that seek to depict a state of mind, a moment of experiencing, are interspersed throughout the book as interludes and examples of Body Words. These interludes are not necessarily tied to the themes of particular chapters. Running through all the chapters are instances of the analyst's use of self.

Chapter 2

In retrospect, it is not surprising that the first paper I published (Chapter 2) is about the body, written in the context of my bout with breast cancer. "When the Analyst Is Ill: Dimensions of Self-Disclosure" examines questions related to the analyst's "inescapable," "inadvertent," and "deliberate" personal disclosures. I explore the technical and personal considerations that influence my decision to disclose, as well as the inherent responsibilities and potential clinical consequences involved. Descriptions of my clinical work during a period of prolonged illness illustrate how self-disclosure may be regarded as both an occasional authentic requirement and a regular intrinsic aspect of clinical technique. In particular, the central clinical vignette anticipates my concept of an *outrageous interpretation*, elaborated in Chapter 6. In the case I describe in Chapter 2, I find myself compelled to deliver from my body a passionate retort to a patient's disavowed hostility. The raw Body Words I spontaneously use serve to punctuate the deadening obstacle of our mutually enacted dissociative avoidance of aggression.

Chapter 3

The title of Chapter 3, "When the Crunch Is a (K)not: A Crimp in Relational Dialogue," employs a pun (*not* and *knot*) to emphasize that a relational (k)not negates truly intersubjective dialogue by shutting down the spaces for mentalization, reflective functioning, genuine affect, and negotiation between and within persons. Between persons, a relational (k)not is a particular entrapping form of disconnect between words deployed at the surface and the affective truths that leak or radiate from the body. Much like the paralyzing contradictions of the "double bind" (Weakland, 1960), the relational (k)nots I describe abort relational freedom (Stern, 2015) and genuine conversation and connection.

In treatment, relational (k)nots appear as repetitions, less heated but more subversive than Russell's (2006a) *crunch* with its intensities of crisis that precipitate greater entanglement. Relational (k)nots instead coerce states of *noninvolvement* between patient and analyst. Persistent relational (k)notting produces a crisis of mutual *detachment*. After offering a developmental perspective on the etiology of relational (k)nots, based on parental failure to mentalize the child's separate subjectivity, I offer an extended clinical vignette to illustrate (k)notting and subsequent disengagement between analyst and patient.

Chapter 4

In Chapter 4, "Passion, Responsibility, and 'Wild Geese': Creating a Context for the Absence of Conscious Intentions," I build on Stephen Mitchell's

(2000) notions of intersubjectivity and the analyst's and patient's separate role responsibilities in the creation of a context for the absence of conscious intention. In this way I introduce my concept of the nonanalytic third and the particular contribution poetry can make to clinical process. I demonstrate how poetry infuses my way of thinking, feeling, and writing and my way of working analytically. A *non*analytic third is the analyst's personal, intimate, and substantially abiding relationship to some body of experience unrelated to *materia psychoanalytica.*

I posit that this nonanalytic third, the nature of which is unique to each analyst, constitutes a source of enrichment, texture, and dimensionality as well as personally compelling metaphors that the analyst may offer to the patient as other-than-me substance. It is also a placeholder for cultivating the potential in the discourse of analytic potential space and serves as a facilitator and comfort for transition when the analyst must recognize and promote the necessary ending of an intimate analytic relationship. These ideas are illustrated with a detailed case example of an unfolding analytic process that includes an e-mail exchange at the time when a shocking form of nonanalytic third appeared—September 11, 2001. As this case demonstrates, a nonanalytic third may become an analytic third.

Chapter 5

Chapter 5, "Narrative Writing and Soulful Metaphors: Commentary on Paper by Barbara Pizer," was written by Donnel B. Stern and published in *Psychoanalytic Dialogues* with "Passion, Responsibility, and 'Wild Geese': Creating a Context for the Absence of Conscious Intentions." Stern focuses on my use of both a narrative and lyrical writing style, which is atypical in the psychoanalytic scholarly tradition. Stern highlights that the nonanalytic third may become a "soulful metaphor" that can be used to create alternatives to rigid experience.

Chapter 6

Chapter 6, "'Eva, Get the Goldfish Bowl': Affect and Intuition in the Analytic Relationship," is an extended clinical narrative that illustrates what I call an *outrageous interpretation*, which takes both analyst and analysand by surprise. In an unexpected moment, I found myself blurting out a reaction to my patient from a dissociated place in me in an implicit effort to make affective contact with a dissociative place in my patient.

In retrospect, an outrageous interpretation can be seen as an attempt to enliven a dead zone between patient and analyst and perhaps make available to each access to defensively walled-off, trauma-related affects, like shame and loneliness.

Chapter 7

Chapter 7, "From Black Hole to Potential Space: Discussion of Barbara Pizer's "'Eva, Get the Goldfish Bowl'": Affect and Intuition in the Analytic Relationship'" was written by Stuart A. Pizer. He elaborates on how an outrageous interpretation may serve to infuse a patient's dissociative black hole with a force of affect that may transform an evacuated space into a potential space.

Chapter 8

Chapter 8, "Risk and Potential in Analytic Disclosure: Can the Analyst Make 'the Wrong Thing' Right?" explores the multiple meanings of analyst disclosures and the application of a fixed analytic frame. I challenge the idea that most analytic rules can universally hold true outside the context of a particular and ever-changing clinical situation. I believe that questions pertaining to "right" and "wrong" are, perhaps, an inapt line of inquiry in this regard. Drawing perspective from reflections on my own developmental history as it relates to disclosure and risk, I describe how these factors play out in the dyadic interactions of a particular, out-of-the-ordinary, highly charged clinical case. I contrast the risks of a potentially inappropriate application of generic analytic rules with the risks and potentials of invoking a personal connection with a hierarchy of ethical principles.

Chapter 9

Chapter 9, "The Heart of the Matter in Matters of the Heart: Power and Intimacy in Analytic and Couples Relationships," is based on the assumption that power and intimacy play a critical role in the development and potential for ongoing growth in both personal and clinical relationships. While defining the distinguishing characteristics of power and intimacy in each context, I propose that in any two-person relationship, analytic or otherwise, the power of intimacy at its best is achieved when there exists a relative balance—acceptable to both participants—in the inevitable dialectic between intimacy and power, a dialectic that cannot remain static and, therefore, requires mutual awareness and tending from moment to moment. Drawing from vignettes extending over decades of marriage and clinical practice, this chapter illustrates ways in which intimacy may flourish or falter in the face of unexamined transferences.

I look primarily at how urgencies related to power may set the power/intimacy dialectic off course and thereby threaten to disrupt either the analytic or personal relationship. Distinguishing between constructive and destructive forms of power, I relate these to intimacy inside and outside the consulting room and offer a clinical example of the impact on the patient when the analyst emerges from behind a string of interpretations. These interpretations speak directly to the patient from his felt experience and thereby open relational space that had been locked shut in impasse.

Chapter 10

"A Clinical Exploration of Moving Anger Forward: Intimacy, Anger, and Creative Freedom," Chapter 10, is an exploration of anger and its potential to impede or facilitate creative or analytic process. Conceptually, I consider anger in terms of cognitive-affective linking and unlinking, with reference to neuroscience research findings, transference-countertransference enactments, and the repetition compulsion as an encoded second language. At its experiential center, this chapter tells the story of a story that could not be told about anger in a distressed clinical process.

Chapter 11

In Chapter 11, "Maintaining Analytic Liveliness: 'The Fire and the Fuel' of Growth and Change," I present the treatment of a man I call Aaren Kahn, who has a prodigious verbal ability, musical talent, and polyglot intellectual interests but, nevertheless, remained affectively inarticulate until we discover a new way of working clinically. Before we made that joint discovery, when Aaren Kahn is still unavailable for relationship, I ask myself how do we locate felt experiencing within ourselves when experiencing within the other is adamantly denied or when the other specifically requests that we do not know what we might know before the other finds it in himself. By eventually linking our talking cure with body-based practices and clinical modalities, this quiet man with a nonverbal quirk, who gave up his wish to play violin in a national orchestra, comes to discover the life within his deadened lexicon.

Chapter 12

"'Trauma, Dissociation, and Disorganized Attachment': A Clinical Collage Engaging Giovanni Liotti's Work," Chapter 12, is written in appreciation of Giovanni Liotti's significant contributions to our understanding of attachment, trauma, and dissociation. I offer the clinical story of a rare patient: a woman who entered treatment as an adolescent, crippled by extraordinary childhood traumas of omission and commission that afflicted her with severe psychological disability. In our more than thirty years of work together, including eventually an analysis, she established a stable independent mode of life and developed creative forms of expression that utilized her giftedness in verbal and musical arts despite testing neurologically as incapable of experiencing vision or hearing. I thereby indicate how an analysis may facilitate a lived life without being a cure-all.

Chapter 13

Drawing on my own experience of sexual abuse decades ago in a first analysis, Chapter 13 reveals the deep and abiding residue that shadows my psyche throughout my life. However, in "'Why Can't We Be Lovers?' When the Price of Love Is Loss of Love: Boundary Violations in Clinical Context," I argue that what we can learn from this must not be reduced to prohibitions and inhibitions that send affects underground, nor prescriptive rules that may shut down an authentic and energized relatedness—in Body Words—between analyst and patient. But, rather, I wish to promote a culture, a climate, and the preparatory conditions to equip clinicians to be competent and clear headed about the powerful affects they permit themselves to feel. I ask: how might we be trained to use ourselves creatively within the conventions and constraints of our school of thought? How and when is love speakable in a clinical context? What role does the transgenerational transmission of trauma play in the way we handle clinical difficulties? Are the therapist's sexual feelings abnormal? How might they be healthily processed? How much do we share with our patients or otherwise express? How do we distinguish between limits and inhibitions? These are just a few of the questions for us to review and revisit again and again.

Chapter 14

In Chapter 14, "Not-Me: The Vicissitudes of Aging," I offer candid vignettes, from the inside out and from the outside in, that exemplify the embodied experiences of aging, especially for women. More generally, I apply Harry Stack Sullivan's (1953) conceptual model of a "self-system" shaped by the reflected appraisals of others and emphasize how the anxieties and reactions of others to external signs of aging may impact a person's ownership and/or defensive dis-ownership ("Not-Me") of her aging self. I offer a concept of "Old-Me," a later-in-life personification that may be "good" or "bad" but provides a more conscious, life-affirming alternative than the dissociative option of "Not-Me." Finally, I recommend and briefly illustrate specific measures a person may deploy to infuse aging with aliveness.

Chapter 15

In this chapter, "Body Words: Transforming the Unspeakable in Clinical Process," I have arrived at the language for my concept of Body Words and explicate how they emerge in clinical process in inverse proportion to the repetition compulsion. So it is that I see the clinician's task in every psychoanalytic treatment as involving a particular focus on the reclamation and growth of the availability of Body Words in both participants, which I illustrate in my work with Doreen. This treatment also demonstrates that the forward movement in therapy can be inhibited, as Paul Russell (2006b) asserts, by the therapist's resistance to what the patient is feeling.

And finally, I outline how my writing—whether daily session notes, associative diary entries, or more formally constructed journal articles—serves a self-supervisory function while also providing a sturdy container for evanescent process moments of Body Words. Once written, Body Words take their place as narrative, reflection, and memory, preserving experience for future reverie or conceptualization.

Chapter 16

Chapter 16 is a coda entitled "Bodies and Embodiment, 1963: The Person of the Analyst." It's an early piece of writing, prior to my psychoanalytic education, manifesting body words and the use of self as I experience my implicatedness during the early sixties' turmoil for civil rights.

The Psyche and the Social

Psychoanalysis is finally beginning to address important relationships between the psyche and the social, the impact of social injustice, and the disparities between classes, races, and genders. As our attention shifts to these issues, my central concept of Body Words and the need to reclaim and develop the accessibility of Body Words in each participant also apply to partners and groups in conflict and conversation outside of our consulting rooms. Because Body Words may emerge in inverse proportion to the repetition compulsion, we need to cultivate the capacity of opposing parties to use them wherever they have been mired in psychological or institutional repetitions.

I hope in future writing to explore the place of Body Words in the service of transforming conversations about race, class, and gender into more genuine dialogue.

References

Gendlin, E. (1962). *Experiencing and the creation of meaning.* Glencoe, IL: The Free Press of Glencoe.

Gendlin, E. (1978). *Focusing.* New York, NY: Random House.

Mitchell, S. A. (2000). *Relationality: From attachment to intersubjectivity.* Hillsdale, NJ: The Analytic Press.

Russell, P. L. (1996). Process with involvement. In L. Lifson (Ed.), *Understanding therapeutic action: Psychodynamic concepts of cure* (pp. 201–216). Hillsdale, NJ: The Analytic Press.

Russell, P. L. (2006a). The theory of the crunch. *Smith College Studies in Social Work,* 76(1/2), 9–21 (written in 1987).

Russell, P. L. (2006b). The role of loss in the repetition compulsion. *Smith College Studies in Social Work,* 76(1/2), 85–98 (written in 1988).

Stern, D. B. (1997). *Unformulated experience: From dissociation to imagination in psychoanalysis.* Hillsdale, NJ: The Analytic Press.

Stern, D. B. (2015). *Relational freedom: Emergent properties of the interpersonal field.* New York, NY: Routledge.

Sullivan, H. S. (1953). *The interpersonal theory of psychiatry.* New York, NY: W.W. Norton & Co.

Weakland, J. H. (1960). The "double bind" hypothesis of schizophrenia and three party interaction. In D. D. Jackson (Ed.), *The etiology of schizophrenia* (pp. 373–388). New York, NY: Basic Books.

Reverie

In the Beginning

Patient

What do you think you are doing, you wonder, as you take the elevator up to the fifth floor where you will meet the person you have chosen for your therapist—possibly your analyst—for the first time. *And what makes you think that she could help you?* All right, so you heard her give a paper a few months ago, you've been considering … and she comes highly recommended. (*Do you think she knows she's highly recommended? And if so, does that make her better or worse for you?*) Will she pay attention—will she really listen? Forget that for a second. What about you? How are you going to say what you have to say when you don't really know the words to find for this uncomfortable gnawing feeling that plagues you just before you open your eyes every morning? And then it goes away as you get into things, but still there is this underneath lingering thing that haunts you for the rest of the day, tugging at you—distracting. But how will you begin to explain it, make yourself understood, and *do you dare?*

Analyst

"So, what brings you here?" she asks, at the same time wondering about that question for herself. *What do I think I'm doing anyway?* Is it bravery or chutzpah that gives me the right to allow a perfect stranger off the street to come into my space with God knows what on her mind—let alone what's going on in her psyche—and me inviting it? I should have my head examined! Forget that for a second. What makes me think I have anything to offer here? How do I dare to begin with this stranger?

DOI: 10.4324/9781032666303-2

Author

And now, as I begin to write my book, reliving these visceral memories from both sides of the couch, once again a fearful uncertainty intrudes. *Who do I think I am?* Come on, that's not true … *What really matters to me is that the essential message carried in this book depends so much on how it is delivered. How will I accomplish what I actually want to do? And what makes that so important?* Forget that. *Will I be able to create a space for the reader to actually enter in and go along until some personal wonder takes its own direction? Will I be able … and do I dare?*

Chapter 2

When the Analyst Is Ill

Dimensions of Self-Disclosure

In a paper entitled "Self-Disclosure: Is It Psychoanalytic?" (1995), Greenberg describes a case in which he elects to meet a patient's repeated question with repeated analytic silence. He cites this vivid instance as an illustration of how and why, in his view, his particular technical choice, with this particular person, in this particular moment bore analytic fruit. Jacobs (1995), in discussing this paper, applauds Greenberg's sensitive treatment, yet goes on to suggest that there *are* times, *some* times, when self-disclosure serves him and his patients well. Along with an increasing number of analysts writing about self-disclosure as potentially useful in furthering the interactive process,[1] Jacobs is careful to say that personal self-disclosure "is quite another, and even more problematic matter" (p. 240). He also asserts that "self-disclosure cannot be prescribed as a general technique" (p. 245). And, along with all of us who wish to keep before us a disciplined awareness of the dangers as well as the benefits inherent in sharing ourselves with those who have put themselves in the patient's position, Jacobs necessarily states the obvious: self-disclosure

> is a delicate matter, one that can do harm as well as possibly prove beneficial. Whether to use it, and in what way, are not easy matters to decide. Such decisions can only be made at a given moment in the clinical situation. (p. 245)

In this chapter I explore these issues raised by Jacobs.

A. What *is* the matter, or what might be the matters involved in personal self-disclosure? What might we make of the consequences of the direct imposition of content from the analyst's personal life upon the patient?

DOI: 10.4324/9781032666303-3

B. Our increasing knowledge of human development as well as our willingness to engage with this matter of self-disclosure suggests that it is indeed a substantial element in our technical considerations. Since such behavior inevitably does depend upon a given moment in the clinical situation—as it depends upon ethics and propriety—it ought to be as speakable in terms of general technique as other topics of controversy such as "interpretation" (Aron, 1992), "resistance" (Bromberg, 1995), or "enactment" (Renik, 1993). Further, I see a greater danger in eschewing discussion of self-disclosure in terms of general technique with the rationalization that new analysts may not be mature enough to utilize such technique. This leaves self-disclosure in the realm of closet activity for the seasoned and a willy-nilly, ill-considered subterfuge on the part of younger colleagues.

C. Hence, this chapter concerns itself with whether or not, or in what way, we might consider personal self-disclosure as speakable among us, as a viable option in a particular clinical moment. Following these points I will consider three aspects of self-disclosure.[2] They are, *as perceived by the analyst*, self-disclosures that are

1. Inescapable
2. Inadvertent
3. Deliberate

I will discuss the first two aspects in relation to my work with patients during a year of sustained illness. The concept of deliberate self-disclosure will be focused on particularly in relation to the "double bind," which I will define as a specific form of resistance as explicated by Bromberg (1995).

Inescapable Self-Disclosure

In the last days of May 1994, four weeks prior to my annual vacation month, a routine mammogram revealed a startling abnormality. With little notice, I would begin my vacation a few weeks earlier to undergo a lumpectomy on the 15th of June and, subsequent to the pathology report, a mastectomy in July. I returned to work at the end, rather than the expected beginning, of August. Chemotherapy began in September of that year and was administered every three weeks for six months. I arranged to have my chemo on Friday afternoons so that the worst of the side effects would abate by Monday when I would be back at work. I rearranged my patient schedule to accommodate one to two hours in the middle of each weekday for rest and meditation. Other than a radical change of hairstyle (very short; I never lost it all) and four unanticipated days out of the office due to a need for a blood transfusion, there were no major disruptions of my schedule. I cannot say the same for the process and content of the work itself. Perhaps my patients would call the term "disruption" an understatement. I told them all I had breast cancer.

This self-disclosure was experienced by me as inescapable. I define inescapable self-disclosure as the analyst's action resulting from the presence in the treatment situation of a circumstantial event whose disruptive properties *in the mind of the analyst* can be handled only by verbal acknowledgment. More simply stated, it is "the elephant in the room" phenomenon.

The circumstantial event may originate in the life of the analyst (e.g., a fire, an illness, or the death of a loved one) or in the patient, as in the case of Donald described by S. Pizer (1992), in which the therapist felt it necessary to say that he was distracted by the effort to tolerate his patient's body odor.

The elements of time and choice distinguish inescapable self-disclosure from inadvertent and deliberate self-disclosure. In contrast to inadvertent self-disclosure, inescapable self-disclosure allows the analyst time to consider what she or he feels must inevitably be said. And in contrast to deliberate self-disclosure, in inescapable self-disclosure the analyst's subjective choice of what and how much must be said is dictated by a particular obtrusive circumstance rather than by the intrinsic clinical process. To reemphasize: the omnipresent threat of disruption is most often the thundercloud contained within an inescapable disclosure. Along with the analyst's awareness of the necessity for some kind of disclosure is the concomitant dread of a subsequent eruption in the analytic interaction.

I emphatically believe that the degree and manner of a self-disclosure by any analyst is, and must always be, inextricably linked to that analyst's conscious and unconscious dynamics.[3] Participation through self-exposure, to whatever degree and whatever the content, is necessarily determined not only by the analyst's technical framework, but by her personal boundaries, beliefs, and sense of comfort. For example, Abend (1982) describes how, upon his return to work after a serious illness, he overrode his determination not to disclose. Responding to persistent inquiries, he did disclose his illness to several patients. Abend then reports his subsequent second thoughts about these disclosures, retrospectively regarding them as unnecessary distractions from the transference implications of his patients' inquiries (see also Dewald, 1982). Many analysts locate their comfort in, and advocate for, keeping their private selves at a distance from the analytic discourse.

Yet another position was bravely taken and bravely reported by Amy Morrison (1997). She continued to see her patients as her own health declined until she died of breast cancer. In her paper she describes how she carefully, selectively, tactfully, and responsibly discussed the reality of her illness with *some* of her patients. Not every therapist with breast cancer would make the personal choice to disclose her condition to her patients. *Nor should she.* Among the many personal issues one may or may not choose to share with a patient, cancer is an intensely personal matter. And a matter of this magnitude—with a course both invisible and invasive, with an outcome at best unpredictable and at worst leading to death—may certainly plunge the person of the analyst into states of uncertainty or anxiety, even terror. While the awareness of uncertainty or anxiety in the analyst will most likely be communicated to one's patients, these raw states—as states in themselves—are problematic when either denied or directly "bled" out into the room. The analyst must find some words to explain and contain these affects, but not necessarily in concrete informational form. For both persons, the stark exposure of the analyst's anxiety surges—specifically about her cancer—can be a mutually destabilizing force that undermines the analytic process in a variety of ways (e.g., the patient may flee, deny his or her senses, or attempt to take care of the analyst). Thus, each analyst must remain attentive and connected to her own sense of how stable she can remain in the face of her uncertainties, how grounded and prepared she is to deal with whatever surprises of affect or inquiry may arise. My own choice to disclose my illness to patients grows out of who I am as a person, and who I am as a practicing clinician.

I will attempt to describe some sense of the self I was aware of when I told my patients that I had breast cancer.

At the most conscious level, I felt a sense of responsibility to disclose—to give my patients maximal opportunity to plan in the face of an unwanted, unpredictable situation; to think about a referral, a consultation, an interruption; to express a variety of feelings at a time when I felt whole, strong, calm, and surprisingly capable. (This is characteristic of my emergency mode.) I hasten to add that this sense of responsibility, this sense of wanting to let my patients in on the beginning in order to maximize their choices of action does not originate in an abstract principle of how one "ought to behave." I have an aversion to out-of-control surprises. When I was a young child, my sister and I were walking home with my mother late one winter night when suddenly she compelled us to run ahead of her. "Run ahead children, *run ahead!*" My mother was unbelievably private about her person and inexpressive in general. It was not usual for her to raise her voice; we had never seen her cry. Now without warning or explanation, she was pushing us away from the comforting presence of her body, shoving us forward into the dark. And then, through the darkness I heard these intense, guttural, wracking sounds and an inexplicable splatter. I felt certain that my mother was being cut apart, and bleeding. Rooted to the spot on the sidewalk to which we had been commanded—too far away from mother— I stamped my feet and wailed through the blackness: "Mommy's dying, Mommy's dying!" "Barbara," said my elder sister who managed upsets with disdain, "Mother is throwing up." (Following this event, our mother took us home and happily informed us over cocoa and cookies that we were going to have a new baby.)

Despite the stresses and shocks of growing up, I am by nature a hopeful person. When the toxicity of chemo did indeed cause cells to die, and I did indeed feel like my life was ebbing away, I nevertheless did not expect to die at this particular time. Further, I did not experience myself as a person who is preoccupied with death. I am more afraid of not fully living in the moment than I am of dying. (I used to say, I am much more afraid of throwing up than of dying, but chemo has cured me of that fear!) There are those who have told me that they have benefited from my "courage"—although "courage" is not my felt experience. If courage is the operative word, then I resonate with it in terms of what for me may be the tributaries of courage: faith and discipline happily augmented by loving support, all of which was available to me before the advent of cancer. I believe that throughout my illness, I could say to myself that I have never felt so sick and so well at the same time.

The more neurotic components of my awareness involved shame, embarrassment, and guilt. (Therapists and mothers betray their contracts when they draw attention to themselves.) Although I would certainly not deny the need for sympathy (see Renik, 1993), I sense that my guilt was the stronger affect. This may have operated in favor of the work; that is to say, when I received sympathy, I was—along with being grateful—hyperalert to what may lie beneath or alongside of it. I was anxious, perhaps overanxious to do the analytic job. I recognized all too well that whatever else my patients and I would be able to make of my inescapable self-disclosure, cancer was and is an invasion of our interaction. At the same time, issues of life and death, change, loss, and grief lie at the center of human experience and growth; and I took hope in the belief that my patients and I could put this inescapable event to analytic use.

I will attempt to highlight some of the interactions stimulated by my self-disclosure. The most common reactions went something like this: "I feel so helpless and so angry about your cancer, and I know it has to do with my parents but..." or simply, "I feel really *bad* about feeling so helpless, and I really don't want you to make anything out of it," or "yes, I'm aware of the transference implications but I'm *so angry!!*" Of course my responses depended upon the person and the moment but in the first instance cited above I did say, "It seems to me that cancer invites both helplessness and anger in both of us, and maybe we should talk about that before we bring your parents into it." In the case of the woman who felt bad about her sense of helplessness and didn't want some "deep interpretation," I replied, "What's to make of it? Here I am telling you my condition and at the same time rejecting your repeated offers of help." As for my response to a patient's somewhat bewildered experience of outrage, I offered the following clarification: "Look, if when you came here five years ago, I gave you the choice of seeing an analyst who would get cancer in five years or someone who wouldn't, which one would you choose? *I* know who *I* would choose!"

Of course, had the clinical situation not been freighted with my illness, my responses to statements of helplessness and anger would have consisted primarily of inquiry. In the first instance, "I wonder what it is now that brings your parents to mind?"; in the second, "Can you say more?" I can imagine meeting the expression of rage with a kind of accepting grunt and waiting for what might follow.

The issue I wish to illustrate and emphasize here is that whenever the analyst feels compelled or chooses (deliberate self-disclosure) to reveal something about herself to a patient, she remains *responsible* for that revelation as she considers every subsequent interaction in the life of that particular treatment. This responsibility implies that the analyst's choice to disclose material from her life must be considered in the light of how much she feels she can burden herself and her patient with the additional complexities of the interactive data. Responsibility implies her effort to remain alert to her shared personal material in the same spirit with which she attempts to follow the development of her patient's material as it manifests itself in the analytic dyad. Today, with some exceptions, I see my patients' anger with me as motivated by more current failures than by the fact that I brought my illness into their lives, but I remain alert to, and prepared for, that possibility. Also, as in other well-worn and speakable elements of discourse, I believe that in general my patients do not shy away from bringing up this unfortunate disruption themselves, particularly around my vacations.

There is another thread in relation to the subject of transference that I do not want to lose. It relates to the paradoxical nature of transference. I am in good company in my belief that every transference is at some level not-transference, and every not-transference is at some level transference (see Ferenczi, 1933; Freud, 1915; Modell, 1991; S. Pizer, 1992). This was cogently illustrated for me by three of my patients just before I left, fifteen days early, for my scheduled vacation. Given the sudden and stark nature of the circumstances, the uncertainties associated with any surgery, and my additional (what I thought would be) four-week absence from the office, I offered patients the option of calling in to ascertain that I was alive and well. Here are examples, albeit stereotypical, where one might possibly entertain the notion that not-transference-transference can manifest itself linguistically in a single word.

My forever-oppressed-by-mother Jewish patient told me that although she most certainly wanted to know how I was, she didn't want to "*intrude*." My stereotypical WASP patient expressed concern that she would "*burden*" me with her needs; a first-generation Chinese-American supervisee feared that a call from her would constitute an "*imposition*." In every one of these cases—"intrude," "burden," and "impose"—the not-transference intention is similar and conveyed: however, we can hypothesize a transferentially unique and distinct cultural and family history embedded in the selective linguistic choice by each of them. As Stuart Pizer (1992) has indicated, "the meaning of language is negotiated in each child-parent dyad" (p. 220).

Inadvertent Self-Disclosure

In her forthright and incisive discussion of Greenberg's paper on self-disclosure, Ehrenberg (1995) concerns herself with countertransference self-disclosure. Her term approximates my notion of inadvertent self-disclosure. Ehrenberg expresses her belief that countertransference disclosure

can help open to analytic scrutiny very subtle dimensions of the analytic field that often might remain inaccessible otherwise. With regard to the latter, my emphasis is not on countertransference disclosure as something to be used as a "parameter" only at moments of impasse or difficulty. My position is more radical. I believe judicious countertransference disclosure has the potential to facilitate a level of analytic engagement and a level of analytic exploration with all patients that may not be possible otherwise. (p. 227)

I am in hearty agreement with Ehrenberg and echo her prescriptions of caution and judiciousness. However, we have a minor and perhaps inconsequential difference, in that she cuts the conceptual cake somewhat differently. We both adhere to the notion that countertransference self-disclosure involves "the analyst's revelation of his or her feelings in *interaction* with the patient or in relation to the patient, at a particular time" (pp. 213-214). But, says Ehrenberg, "I distinguish this from any number of other forms of disclosure. The latter can range from revealing information about ourselves, such as details of our personal history, where we go on vacation, [etc.]" (p. 214).

Here Ehrenberg *sections off process from content.* I am less able or inclined to make the cut between these two. There are disclosures that extend beyond reporting to the patient how the patient's transference is making the analyst feel in the countertransference. Given the complexity of therapist-patient dynamics, I do not want to draw so sharp a line between process and content. So often *process is a content and content is a process.*

I illustrate with an example from my own experience outside of the consulting room. (This is a deliberate self-disclosure.) Take the content, "I hate crows." Innocuous enough. Remember, then, or extrapolate from what I have already indicated, that I knew very little about my mother's internal processing other than her incredible efforts to be a "correct mother." One fall morning, much later in our lives, when we both knew that Alzheimer's was increasingly loosening my mother's fine mind, we were walking together in a beautiful meadow-like garden rimmed with the crimson foliage of the season. But it felt like summer still, the sky was very clear and blue, the songs of birds were amplified, and a light breeze played around our ankles. My mother turned to me, looked me straight in the eye, and said, "I hate crows."

Today, as well as then, I cling to that piece of information as to a talisman. Without a doubt, this expression, this particular articulation of a strong and clear feeling delivered to me by my mother in this moment of our lives, constituted a marker: the beginning of a healing of childhood terror and uncertainty over what my mother might suddenly emit. Aron (1992), in a paper called "Interpretation as Expression of the Analyst's Subjectivity," broadens the definition of interpretation as a "reciprocal communication process." He writes:

> An interpretation has impact on the one giving it as well as the one receiving it. That is one reason, when a patient interprets to the analyst, it may be of benefit not only to the analyst but to the patient as well, and vice versa. (p. 502)

The interaction between my mother and myself provided a content that is not merely informational, in the sense that she was also metaphorically interpreting something for us both. We both came to understand that she put her reality into her feeling about the squawking of crows—a reality that penetrated through our atmosphere. All her life she would rather die (and she, also, was not afraid of dying) than make a noise. Commotion repelled her. And I have been able to use, in a Winnicottian sense, the moment in which she told me all about that in three words, "I hate crows." As Aron, describing Winnicott, writes, "interpretation may be useful not because it provides new information (content) but rather because it represents a link with the analyst (process) ... [that] can be carried around ... when the analyst is away" (p. 485). Aron (along with others—Ferenczi, Hoffman, Renik) states that every intervention or nonintervention discloses something about the analyst. It is from his work that I draw my notion of inadvertent self-disclosure. He writes: "Inadvertent self-revelation is inevitable, and in addition, I do believe that there are many times when direct expression of the analyst's experience is useful" (p. 481).

In his discussion, Aron makes a valuable contribution toward clarifying the various and necessarily idiosyncratic stances taken by contemporary analysts. Rather than cutting up the cake one way or another, Aron provides us with dimensions and degrees of freedom. On one continuum he postulates a mutuality-non-mutuality dimension, and on another, a symmery-asymmetry dimension. Mutuality-nonmutuality refers to the degree to which the analyst recognizes "the reciprocal influence that patient and analyst have on each other," while symmetry-asymmetry refers to "the division of responsibility in the dyad" (p. 482). Seeing himself as radical on the mutuality-nonmutuality dimension (his theoretical and clinical conception of the transference-countertransference matrix) and favoring moderate asymmetry (what the analyst is and is not free to say) Aron (1992) writes:

> Analysts should be cautious in regard to self-revelations, for they are always complicated and problematic; however, everything that the analyst says or does not say is complicated and problematic. What is critical is not whether the analyst chooses to reveal something at a particular moment to a patient, but, rather, the analyst's skill at utilizing this in the service of the analytic process. Is the analyst, or, more accurately put, is the particular analyst-patient dyad able to make use of the analyst's self-revelation in the service of clarifying and explicating the nature of their interaction? In other words, does this intervention lead to further analysis of the transference-countertransference? (p. 483)

I will return to this particular quotation later on, but for the moment I wish to define inadvertent self-disclosure as an inevitable outcome of the analyst's active engagement with a patient. Such self-disclosures may or may not contain within them elements from the analyst's life experience. The responsible analyst, with appropriate caution, and respect for the power inherent in any self-disclosure on her part, must be prepared for this eventuality. Inadvertent self-disclosure requires, above all else, the analyst's skill in utilizing the potential of the shared contents of her experience in the service of the analytic process.

Inadvertent Self-Disclosure: Case Illustration

Dr. T is the eldest daughter of a large well-to-do family dominated by a narcissistic, neurasthenic, alcoholically unpredictable mother who delegated Dr. T as a caretaker of her siblings as well as of mother herself in her various moods of exaltation or despair. Promised rewards of special luncheons out or shopping expeditions were more often than not rescinded because mother would claim headaches or some "fatigue" of unknown origin. Even before my illness, Dr. T and I were not surprised by her incredible vigilance over my states of being. We knew that, for her, any distractions or discomforts on my part would be perceived as signals to negate her needs and to tend to mine. Dr. T has required much of me over the years. But one of her most impressive characteristics is the unflinching and persistent way in which she has required equally as much of herself. She does not spare herself. On days that she would rather do anything else than come to analysis to face our work, she drags herself in to pursue it. Throughout the stormiest of times she has never let me lose sight of her integrity. Over the years, my admiration for this woman's relentless quest for herself has deepened into love.

On this Monday morning she came into the office and, rather than taking up where we had left off on the Thursday before, she sat down in an uncharacteristic manner, assuming a body position that I had come to associate with her sense of unarticulated outrage. Although she did not say so, I suspected she somehow knew I'd had my chemo on the previous Friday. She asked me how I was, and I answered, "Pretty good, thanks." There followed a long silence. Then, sitting back, she spoke in an unusually soft and solicitous tone: "I am not going to sit here and tell you what's going on inside of me. How can I? I bring in ordinary, run-of-the-mill issues, and you bring cancer. I'm not," she said softly, "going to tell you how I am in pain." At that, I discovered myself leaning forward in my chair and in a tone also uncharacteristically low, but fairly spitting out the words, I heard myself saying, "I have lost a breast. Now do you want to take my milk away from me too?" The acknowledgments that followed opened the way to our better understanding (through our experience in the interaction) of how each of us responded to her distrust of women (now speakable between us) as well as to the hostility that accompanies her expectation of abandonment. In my efforts to provide a safe place in which Dr. T might open and deepen an exploration of her desires, I had neglected a crucial aspect of her person. At last she "upped the ante" in such a way that I could no longer avoid talking back to her rage. It would be nice to be able to report that we were both cured—that I no longer slip into the "correct mother" role and that she is now at home in her desires and aggression. But though she may not remember this moment in our time together (she may hold another moment), for me it is an important marker, a moment in which we broke through a critical resistance.

Resistance and the Double Bind: Case Continued

In his paper, "Resistance, Object-Usage, and Human Relatedness," Bromberg (1995) develops his concept of resistance as "an enacted dialectical process of meaning construction, rather than an archeological barrier preventing the surfacing of disavowed reality" (p. 173). Elaborating further, Bromberg describes the motivation of resistance as "not simply an avoidance of insight or fear of change but as a dialectic between preservation and change—*a basic need* to preserve the continuity of self-experience in the process of growth by minimizing the threat of potential traumatization" (p. 174 emphasis added).

Retrospectively, I can see how Dr. T and I had caught ourselves up in a double bind resistance, a repetition of an external and internal state of affairs that characterized Dr. T's (and also my) growing up. I propose that the double bind is a particularly recalcitrant, knotted form of resistance, one in which there is as yet no room to move, no potential for dialectic, no space for negotiation, and hence no growth or change.

We have come to apply the term "double bind" (see Weakland, 1960) to a situation in which a usually less powerful individual is inescapably caught in an intense relationship with another person who is delivering two orders of message, one of which negates the other—messages which deny the possibility of any kind of dialectic. As a consequence, options are perceived as black or white alternatives in a lose-lose situation. (My troubles are nothing compared to yours, so I am silenced. If I talk to you, I'm bad, and you scoff; if I don't, I'm abandoned and alone.)

The quintessential instance: as an adolescent Dr. T was offered the opportunity to escape the overexciting, unpredictable, tyrannical atmosphere of home by going to boarding school, but only under the condition that she get rid of her beloved, but aging and mangy dog, her faithful friend since childhood. She could not bear the conflict and moved to act almost immediately. Her mother promised to stand by her, to help her with her loss, to be with her when she put the dog to sleep. Dr. T reports this interlude as one of their most intimate times. Sitting together then over the dead dog, mother confides for the first time that Dr. T was an unwanted child, conceived out of wedlock, and the reason for her unhappy parents' marriage. She is alive and unwanted, and her dog is dead and wanted, and her mother is in charge of both.

It is no wonder that Dr. T's neediness and rage were so bound up together that she would consistently punish herself for her desires and expect to fail in close relationships. In our interaction I became so concerned about not repeating history with her that, even before my illness, when I had to cancel appointments, I would offer other times, including evenings or weekends. So it was that my overdetermined compliance served to close off from her a space in which to make legitimate protest. I tightened the knot of her double bind rather than opening a potential space in which she could first experience and then begin to traverse the rifts between her love and her hate, her desires and her angers with me.[4]

Once the double bind is loosened, made explicit, or articulated, once there is some provision of space, resistance can become, as Bromberg (1995) writes,

> a "marker" that structures the patient's effort to arrive at new meaning without disruption of self-continuity during the transition, and gives voice to opposing realities within the patient's inner world that are being enacted in the intersubjective and interpersonal field between analyst and patient. (p. 174)

In its foreclosure of that dialectical space described by Bromberg, wherein resistance may be negotiated, the double bind may be considered a preresistance resistance!

Although I had certainly argued with Dr. T, held firm in our transference-countertransference struggles, I had not yet been able to disentangle my own rage from my caring and present it to Dr. T in such a way that we would both have the space, first to perceive and differentiate, and then to bridge these affects within and between us. Subsequent to my inadvertent self-disclosure inspired by Dr. T, we developed our capacity to accommodate the simultaneity of love and hate both internally and externally as these affects occurred in our interaction.

Deliberate Self-Disclosure and Conclusion

Now I believe that Aron would have no quarrel with my inadvertent self-disclosure. I have indicated his position that "self-expression" has a central part in analysts' interpretations which are codetermined. However, Aron (1992) unequivocally states that for

> the analyst deliberately to work his or her way into an interaction with a patient ... would be to interfere with whatever kind of interaction the patient is trying to create. The only legitimate interaction that the analyst should be trying to work his or her way into is that of understanding the meanings of the interaction. (p. 493)

Aron goes on to assert, "Of course *inadvertently* the analyst will *be pulled* into other interactions or enactments ... and will *unwittingly* attempt to push the patient into particular patterns of enactment" (p. 493, emphasis added).

Recall Aron's statement, quoted earlier, that analysts "should be cautious in regard to self-revelations, for they are always complicated and problematic," but, then again, "however, everything that the analyst says or does not say is complicated and problematic" (p. 483).

I want to hold myself more responsible and in control than this. *I believe that there are moments in the clinical process in which the patient indicates a need or a ripeness to receive, for personal use, some elements from the analyst's subjectivity.* That is, the analyst deliberately exercises her clinical judgment that the patient seeks—whether implicitly or explicitly—a sample of how the analyst's separate mind works (associatively, metaphorically, conceptually, etc.) (see Renik, 1995). For example, I believe that there are times when a patient asks the analyst what she is thinking and that the patient is not necessarily occupied or concerned with the impression she is having on the analyst. Sometimes the patient is so knotted in her head— often experienced as a sense of emptiness or nothingness or "drawing a blank"—that she is asking the analyst to offer some "other-than-me substance" (see Winnicott, 1990/1969) that serves to open a space that analytic silence may not, in that instance, provide.

Once when asked that question, I replied, "I'm hearing the sound of the siren outside, and it is reminding me of the distant sound of a train whistle. I am remembering that as a child in bed at night this sound was the loneliest sound in the world." The patient considered this and was able then to go on with her deliberation of a particular issue—experiencing then an unheard of possibility. Ultimately, she said to me, "Do you realize, Barbara, that in all my growing up, I *never* realized that I could resent my mother and love her at the same time. I've been trying so hard to get rid of my resentment."

This put me in mind of my own mother. Toward the end of her life, there was another incident that took place in the night. It was the middle of the night, and I found her wandering through the house in her nightgown, lost, bewildered, and terribly embarrassed. Accompanied by her profuse apologies, I led her back to her room and, soothing, sang her the lullaby she sang to me when I was a child. But now that I had something more of her apart from me, I could accommodate a range of simultaneous feelings that provided a deeper, sturdier, less idealized sense of who each of us was. (I recognize that I strive for this in the work I do with patients.) Now I could let my mother go. Sitting there with her, once again in the darkness, singing her to sleep, I experienced three feelings all at the same time, and they welled up in a kind of concurrent dialogue. I thought, or rather felt, "What a privilege to be able to provide for you in your final time"; and "I guess the best that I can get from you is to give it"; and "*where in God's name were you* when I needed you so badly?" Three feelings—gratitude, acceptance, and rage—all at the same time.

But back to my response to the patient who asked me what I was thinking—and the sound of the train in the night. Mine was not an inadvertent self-disclosure. Perhaps this is dancing on the head of a pin, but I view Aron as conflating inescapable and inadvertent self-disclosure, and if he does tell a patient something from his life, he believes it is because he could not help it: an inevitable (albeit necessary) part of complicated and problematic work. Whereas Ehrenberg (countertransference self-disclosure) separates self-disclosure contents from the analyst's life, from process comments regarding the analyst's feelings in the life of the analytic dyad, Aron tells us (self-expression in the context of "relational perspectivism") that self-expressive contents are unavoidable (or inescapable) *but* should be delivered inadvertently.[5]

Hence, the analyst's contents are still inextricably linked to the analytic process that originates with the patient, thus leaving the analyst—if she believes it serves a purpose—no conscious legitimate recourse to draw from her own distinctly separate life experience.

To my way of thinking, deliberate self-disclosure may not necessarily constitute a boundary violation any more than some other intervention might (see McLaughlin, 1995); as a matter of fact, it may be delivered in a manner that is more respectful of a patient's boundaries. Self-disclosure is not synonymous with mutual analysis (see Dupont, 1985). Aron's (1992) suggestion that "participation should be done inadvertently *as much as possible* [emphasis added] as a response to the patient rather than as a deliberate provocation" (p. 493) does not satisfy my particular need for more clarity in this matter. I conceive of the necessary asymmetry between analyst and patient less in terms of self-disclosure and more in terms of disciplined and responsible behavior (see B. Pizer, 1994; McLaughlin, 1995). There are times in my work with patients when I may speak a content from my life experience not because it is unavoidable, not because I inadvertently let it slip, but because, having considered it, I believe it might contribute, or indeed *open,* the intrapsychic spaces within and the intersubjective spaces between us, thereby extending the potential for movement, for growth, for further dialectic, and ultimate termination.

This chapter, a deliberate self-disclosure, is offered in that spirit.

Notes

1 Among many authors who have considered the issue of self-disclosure, Ferenczi stands out as a pioneer. More recently Aron, Burke, Bollas, Ehrenberg, Hoffman, Maroda, Mitchell, Tansey, Renik, and others have contributed to the literature on this issue.
2 Obviously, these aspects of self-disclosure overlap in actual clinical process, and my own particular system of conceptualizing these component dimensions of a total process, as with any conceptual system, is arbitrary. But I believe that the mental discipline inherent in utilizing a systematic approach (despite its inevitable shortcomings) serves the function of "checks and balances" on the necessarily intuitive and authentic responsiveness of the analyst engaged in the current of a clinical moment.
3 Renik (1995) emphasizes that "an analyst's personality is constantly revealed, *in one form or another*, through his or her analytic activities" (p. 469).
4 Another way of conceiving of this might be in terms of "avoiding the negative transference." Space does not permit detailing in this chapter the distinctions between these two concepts. Suffice it to say that in this case, I perceive my "correct behavior," my cutting her off with kindness, so to speak, as more closely related to our transference-countertransference double bind.
5 Since my writing of this chapter, Aron has continued to develop his own ideas on these issues. For a more current sense of his thinking, see Chapters 7 and 8 in his book, *A Meeting of Minds: Mutuality in Psychoanalysis* (Hillsdale, NJ/London: The Analytic Press, 1996).

References

Abend, S. M. (1982). Serious illness in the analyst: Countertransference considerations. *Journal of the American Psychoanalytic Association, 30*, 365–379.

Aron, L. (1992). Interpretation as expression of the analyst's subjectivity. *Psychoanalytic Dialogues, 2*, 475–507.

Bromberg, P. M. (1995). Resistance, object-usage, and human relatedness. *Contemporary Psychoanalysis, 31*, 173–191.

Dewald, P. A. (1982). Serious illness in the analyst: Transference, countertransference, and reality responses. *Journal of the American Psychoanalytic Association, 30*, 347–363.

Dupont, J. (Ed.). (1985). *The clinical diary of Sándor Ferenczi* (M. Balint & N. Z. Jackson, Trans.). Cambridge, MA: Harvard University Press, 1988.

Ehrenberg, D. B. (1995). Self-disclosure: Therapeutic tool or indulgence? Countertransference disclosure. *Contemporary Psychoanalysis, 31*, 213–228.

Ferenczi, S. (1933). Confusion of tongues between adults and the child. The language of tenderness and of passion. In *Final contributions to the problems and methods of psycho-analysis* (pp. 156–167). New York: Brunner/Mazel, 1980.

Freud, S. (1915). Observations on transference-love. (Further recommendations on the technique of psycho-analysis III. pp. 157–171). *S.E., 12*.

Greenberg, J. (1995). Self-disclosure: Is it psychoanalytic? *Contemporary Psychoanalysis, 31*, 193–211.

Jacobs, T. J. (1995). Discussion of Jay Greenberg's paper. *Contemporary Psychoanalysis, 31*, 237–245.

McLaughlin, J. T. (1995). Touching limits in the analytic dyad. *Psychoanalytic Quarterly, 64*, 433–465.

Modell, A. (1991). The therapeutic relationship as paradoxical experience. *Psychoanalytic Dialogues, 1*, 13–28.

Morrison, A. (1997). Ten years of doing psychotherapy while living with a life threatening illness: Self-disclosure and other ramifications. *Psychoanalytic Dialogues*, *7*, 225–241.

Pizer, B. (1994, April 16). The analyst's countertransference: Use and abuse of intimacy and power. Presented at the spring meeting, Division of Psychoanalysis, American Psychological Association, Washington, DC.

Pizer, S. (1992). The negotiation of paradox in the analytic process. *Psychoanalytic Dialogues*, *2*, 215–240.

Renik, O. (1993). Countertransference enactment and the psychoanalytic process. In M. J. Horowitz, O. F. Kernberg & E. M. Weinshel (Eds.), *Psychic structure and psychic change: Essays in honor of Robert S. Wallerstein, M.D* (pp. 137–160). Madison, CT: International Universities Press.

Renik, O. (1995). The ideal of the anonymous analyst and the problem of self-disclosure. *Psychoanalytic Quarterly*, *64*, 466–495.

Weakland, J. H. (1960). The "double-bind" hypothesis of schizophrenia and three party interaction. In D. D. Jackson (Ed.), *The etiology of schizophrenia* (pp. 373–388). New York: Basic Books.

Winnicott, D. W. (1990/1969). The use of an object and relating through identifications. In *Playing and reality* (pp. 86–94). New York: Basic Books, 1971.

Reverie

A True Story

A true story, you may well know it.[1]

Some years ago in New York City, a young boy was walking home in the early dark of a winter's evening holding a stick outstretched in his right hand. The way he handled the thing like a part of himself, it could have been a champion's tennis racket or policeman's club that brought up confidence or courage as he ambled through the shadowy streets brandishing his stick around, whacking every lamppost that he passed. It seems to me the sound of each substantial whack provided momentary mastery as he held his lonely conversation with the night.

Whack, whack, WHACK!!

Then suddenly, with uncanny precision, he whacked a post, *and the entire city went black!*

Yes, it was the night of the New York Blackout—leaving this young boy reeling in terror and shock and shame because he *knew* that he alone was the source and the victim of a terrible catastrophe . . .

How would he, his loved ones, and his shattered world ever recover from his secret shameful deed?

Note

1 On November 9, 1965, at 5:27 p.m., a blackout occurred as several Northeastern states and part of Canada were hit by a series of power failures lasting as long as thirteen hours. The blackout covered 80,000 square miles and affected more than thirty million people.

   Striking at the evening rush hour, the power failures trapped 800,000 riders on New York City subways. Railroads halted. Traffic was jammed. Airplanes found themselves circling, unable to land. (Reported in *The New York Times*.)

DOI: 10.4324/9781032666303-4

Chapter 3

When the Crunch Is a (K)not
A Crimp in Relational Dialogue[1]

Defining the Terms: The Crunch and the (K)not and Modes of Involvement in Relational Dialogue

In an early paper, Paul Russell (2006a) concerns himself with two dimensions of the treatment process: the repetition compulsion and containment. Russell defines the "crunch" as a particular, inevitable, and necessary crisis in treatment. It is the patient's attempt, often a last-ditch effort, to recreate in the present the traumas or derailments of the past. Inexplicably, the past is catapulted into the consulting room as a threat, a dare, a defiant plea that the therapist do something about which the patient is certain nothing can be done. It is now or never. And if not now, this charade called therapy is over. Russell emphasizes that crunches strain and shake the sanity of the therapist and "all sorts of nutty things tend to happen" (p. 14).

The nutty things that happen have to do with the therapist's unwitting involvement in the patient's repetition and her often engaging in repetitions of her own. Another way of describing the crunch is as a kind of confusion of time, space, and relationship in which it is unclear who is who and what is happening and when—a condition of interpersonal chaos rather than containment. In this boundless predicament, one finds it difficult to step back, to find a way to straddle those "essential paradoxes" described by Russell (2006b) that "surround and invest every repetition" and are implicated in the development of affective competence. Among them are such questions as "Is this me or is this you?" "Is this now or was it then?" "Did I do this or was it done to me?" (p. 96).

The crunch is, to say the least, an affectively laden, if not overloaded, exchange of enactments between two people, a desperate engagement

DOI: 10.4324/9781032666303-5

that carries both a plea for attachment and a despairing certainty that attachments can never be realized. Russell (2006a), however, insists, "if the treatment process has a chance to develop, *every patient will deliver into it their own particular kind of crunch*" (p. 11, emphasis added). And we know that if the treatment process is to succeed, the therapist must find a way to extricate herself from involvement in the patient's repetition and thereby provide the potential for containment, a new experience, and new growth.

In a much later paper, Russell (1996), continuing the idea of the necessary and potentially mutative crunch, describes this crisis as it is delivered into the treatment situation:

> It consists of the patient's delivering something very similar to the repetitive destructive patterns that have occurred before in his life, and which becomes in the process of the negotiation of the treatment process, *a crisis of attachment* involving both patient and therapist. (p. 214)

Developing his ideas from earlier works, Russell (1996) states that the crunch, or the "rendering of the repetition," as he refers to the crisis of engagement, precipitates two risks: The first is that the disaster that created the original anguish will once more occur; and the second is that it will not. He writes, "The rendering of the repetition will powerfully deliver to the therapist every conceivable . . . invitation to be someone other than a therapist" (p. 215). The therapist is urged to enact pieces of relational pattern in the patient's history and is pulled toward enacting those antiquated and stored-away repetitions that stem from vulnerabilities rooted in her own childhood experience. Emphasizing that the treatment process is one of mutual understanding and discovery, Russell continues:

> It is the patient's discovery of who the therapist is, *as therapist*, that connects directly with the second great risk of the treatment process. It is precisely that discovery that gives words, gives feeling to all of the ways in which this experience was not there before, the ways in which what happened before was different. The repetition compulsion is an attempt to coerce identity. The technique of therapy consists of the therapist's being able to survive the attempt at coerced identity and emerge as in fact different. (p. 215)

Good therapy or analysis provides a crucible for emotional growth. It puts *both participants* in touch with a pain that they have not felt before, a pain that enables *memory* as opposed to repetition—a lost memory or memory of loss, loss of what once was or should have been and was not, memories that must be borne and grieved. (If this was me, then that was you. If I open up to the way you were with me, what does that do to our attachment? If I claim who I am, do I lose you? If I lose you, then how do I go on?) For the person sitting in the analyst's place, the capacity to contain and negotiate the treatment process requires, as Russell (1996) emphasizes, *involvement*. The analyst's involvement with "who the *patient* is, with who he is as he is with the patient, and with what is now *happening*, most especially between them . . . takes work. The hardest part is the pain. The pain of memory" (p. 215).

Russell concludes,

> The technique I have found, if I can call it that, is to try to know the time and the place where I become uninvolved. The most dangerous part of the treatment process is when both parties wish for, invite, non-involvement. That is the most dangerous repetition. (pp. 215–216)

We might surmise that the noninvolvement Russell describes has to do with the potential consequences of too much affect in the consulting room. I mean here, however, to identify a particular situation, a microprocess related to the crunch, that silently dictates disengagement, a kind of petrified distortion from the past that enters present dialogue and contributes to what I have come to call a relational (k)not. A (k)not may originate in the earliest relationship between caregiver and infant wherein negating or nonrecognizing messages are preverbally absorbed. Later these messages are encoded and elaborated in procedural memory as habits of mind that exist outside awareness and are as much taken for granted as the very breath of life. When the crunch is a (k)not, or a series of (k)nots leading up to a crunch, a particular crimp in relational dialogue occurs, a negating of space and involvement and therefore a negating of the actual current relationship.

In the title of this chapter, *(k)not* is a play on the word *knot* (see Laing, 1970), which refers to that form of relational dialogue that subverts authentic, open communication. As a consequence, the apparent dialogue presents merely an *image* of two people in conversation: What one person is really saying remains unspoken, and the other person's response—if not already scripted—becomes distorted. Recognition, acknowledgment, and genuine affect necessarily drop out. Without a true dialogical space in this relationship, internal reflection, the capacity for mentalization, is compromised; the possibilities for negotiation between participants are diminished, knotted up, or nullified (see S. Pizer, 1992, 1998). Informed by the double-bind construct originally coined to describe the etiology of schizophrenia in family discourse (Weakland, 1960), I use the term relational (k)not(s) to describe a crimping form of communication that occurs between and within persons along the entire spectrum, from pathology to health, from notably disturbed to relatively well-functioning people.

Crimps in Relational Dialogue: An "Ordinary" Illustration

Let us take a look at a not-unusual conversation between Mother and Daughter, a well-known social psychologist. We may assume that Mother's lifelong depression and inconsistent caregiving have contributed to Daughter's efforts to please her, to get Mother's attention and approval. Professional praise for Daughter's recently published paper, "The Effects of Peer Relations on Learning among Third-World Children in Secondary Schools," seems somehow hollow, and Daughter has given Mother the paper for comment and opinion.

Mother says, "Wonderful paper, dear, very nice job."

Daughter's rejoinder is, "Is that all you have to say?"

Mother answers, "Well . . . Well, I know I'm not as intelligent as one of your Ecuadoran seventh graders in the study, but is there a reason why you persist in using dashes where commas would do?"

Daughter shrugs this off. When Mother turns back to her knitting, Daughter tells Mother how widely the paper has been distributed—in South America and even in Asia.

"Chile to China isn't very far alphabetically," says Mother, continuing to knit.

Daughter gets up to leave the room.

"Where are you going?" asks Mother. The knitting needles suddenly cease clicking. "I thought we were having a conversation!"

Daughter returns to sit in the chair opposite her mother. She pauses for a moment, takes a breath. And then says, "What did you mean when you said the thing about Chile to China?"

The needles resume clicking.

"Mom," Daughter says, more slowly now, quavering but deliberate, "you really hurt my feelings."

Mother tosses her knitting on the coffee table and bursts into tears. "You never hear me when I praise you! I told you nice job! When are you ever going to forget I was a bad mother!"

How might we disentangle this communication? It takes place on at least two levels: the spoken and the unspoken. And within the spoken, messages ricochet between simple concrete statements and higher-order abstractions faster than the speed of light. The dialogue is knotted. Mother begins her sentence by reporting her IQ as below seventh-grade level and, without skipping a beat, becomes a seventh-grade teacher issuing a pedantic comment about improper punctuation. But looking in from the outside, we immediately see clearly that mother is not talking about her daughter's writing style.

We might hypothesize the following: Directly below the surface of mother's blandly uttered inquiry, it is possible to hear the accusation— "I may be stupid, but you are not so smart either." And below that: "I know you look down on me, but I am still your mother, and whatever you bring me, we will, *you* will, engage with me on *my* terms or not at all. But you are stuck with me. Hard as you try, you have no way out."

For example, when Daughter attempts to move the conversation from grammar to a higher level of abstraction, Mother veers back to geography and spelling (Chile and China). And when Daughter tries, literally, to leave the arena, Mother reels her back with the implication that Daughter is either rude or oversensitive. But when Daughter makes a last-ditch effort to voice her pain directly, Mother ups the ante, accusing Daughter now of insensitivity, cinching the relational (k)not with the unspoken, "I may be a bad mom, but you are a worse daughter by not letting me forget it for a moment." What began on the surface as a double bind has ended in a double knot—a relational (k)not.

From the conversation between Mother and Daughter, we are left to wonder, "Is this moment now or was it then?" But we can wonder only from the outside looking in. There is no relational space between the participants themselves. Looking in from the outside, we can imagine Mother preoccupied with her own ungrieved maternal relationship, an insecure, unsatisfying, ambivalent attachment, now projected onto Daughter. We can imagine the crimping consequences of this mother's developmental history, which still leaves her feeling inadequate, insecure, unintelligent, and envious.

We can wonder if Daughter will ever find the space to reflect on why she challenges her mother to say more about the paper. After all, she must *know* her mother by now. Perhaps she is still pursuing the question, "Did I do this, or was it done to me?" And might we not surmise that Mother's legacy of engagement only on her terms, or not at all, has passed through herself to Daughter, who is now stuck in that crimp? At the moment, the daughter's only way out, as far as we can see, is not to think about what just happened, but perhaps to laugh about it, to tell the story to her friends, to dissociate the feelings that her mother has evoked. So what seems to us, on the outside, to be a rather dramatic dialogue, a painful interaction all around, becomes a kind of funny story, a routine, ordinary in the minds of the participants, who are unable to reflect on it. Happens all the time.

Crimps in the Consulting Room

Inevitably, relational (k)nots appear as repetitions in the treatment situation. But the repetition I refer to here is not the *content* of a particular interaction, but the *process*; *a process of uninvolvement*; a process that consists of the "(k)notting" or negating of the original anguish or affect and is, therefore, *not* "rendered" for negotiation between patient and analyst. A relational (k)not, a crimp in thinking, feeling, or interacting, coerces noninvolvement. Persistent relational (k)notting produces a crisis of *detachment* involving both participants. We might see it as the negative or underside of a crunch, wherein genuine affect is subtly, imperceptibly dropped out. The relational (k)not deletes relational space. Whereas a crunch consists of a confusion of time, a foreclosure of space in the relationship between two people, the (k)not conflates time and space and erases relationship. Here is a hypothetical example of a series of interconnecting (k)nots from the consulting room:

> "I don't want an antidepressant because if all it takes is a little pill, then I should be able to do it myself."

Something is missing in that thought process, but it's hard to figure out exactly what. And then—

"If it turns out that I feel better on your pills, then I'll really be upset that I didn't take them sooner!"

How did that happen? The therapist reorients, attempts to grab at the lost stitch. "*My* pills?"

"You know what I mean, the antidepressants."

"*Forget it!*" thinks the therapist to herself, and then the intensity of that instruction is almost imperceptibly replaced by "It's best to let that go for now; it will come up again."

We might infer from this example that there may be something in the patient-person's past that coerces him to assume a correlation between the size or sign of an antidepressant pill and the size or sign of his ability for manly accomplishment. And furthermore, there is something in the past or present situation that causes a particular vulnerability to a perception of coercion; but he is unable to think so or say so directly. And what about the therapist-person's state of awareness? Might her past contain a fear of assertion? Does the presence of latent anger or detachment frighten, or anger, her? What do we have to go on? The repetitions here consist of interlocking instances of dialogical crimps that make up a series of relational (k)nots. There is a jamming of relational space. Sometimes these (k)nots will silently, subversively evade or negate involvement until patient and therapist terminate—both wondering what they somehow left out or missed, and why a pretty good experience did not seem good enough. The relational (k)not is a drag on the necessary crunch; both in its outrageous and its subtle forms, it pulls for disengagement, noninvolvement.

Let us illustrate with an outrageous hypothetical example. A person sitting in the patient's place remarks offhandedly that the charge for a therapy hour comes close to what he would have to pay for a good whore, "Only with a whore you get to do what you want. But, then again, you might not learn as much about yourself." *Now* what happens to the person sitting in the therapist's place? What next?

Russell (1996) tells us that "therapy attempts to understand affect. We try to make sense of what we are feeling" (p. 206). But, here, if the patient has grasped the analyst's particular sensitivities, a particular vulnerability to being called a whore, we can see how the relational (k)not perverts affect. Hence, the identity that is coerced is a dissociated identity. The "nutty thing" that happens is that one's capacity for reflective functioning is severely threatened. What happens to affect?

I am reminded of standing in the crush of a crowded New York subway in rush hour. I perceive something rubbing up against my leg. The man closest to me is concentrated on reading his newspaper. What do I do? Do I say to this man, "Cut it out!" And he retorts, "What are you talking about?" And I say to him, "Quit rubbing at my leg," and he says, "Are you crazy? I'm not doing anything. I'm reading my paper, lady." *You can't fight it and there is no way out.* Something is rubbing your leg, and you can't move. So you detach. What is happening is "not"! You can't confront it, and you can't get away from it. It feels as if survival requires not doing and not being. The original affect is dropped out; the experience is dissociated.

Let's say the patient whose therapist may have smilingly absorbed his high-class-woman-of-the-street analogy might, with sudden surprise, find *himself* out on the street five minutes before the end of his session. In the next session, his therapist may apologize for her oversight; she might suggest that she did not realize her clock was running fast. And so the plot cannot thicken because the knot gets tighter. There is less and less room to face down those paradoxical questions that Russell (2006b) cites as essential to the growth of human feelings, "the paradoxes which point to precisely where the person was [originally] injured" (p. 95) and what it is that he must repeat in the crunch if ever he is to grieve his losses, if ever he can hope for genuine attachment. In the (k)not, these questions are squeezed out or cannot be asked:

"Is this me or is this you?"
"I'm just reading my paper, lady!"
"Did I do this, or was it done to me?"
"Sorry, my clock was running fast."
"Is this now, or was it then?"
"When are you ever going to forget I was a bad mother?"

And there is one more essential paradox that Russell (2006b) asks us to consider: "Can I choose what I feel?" (p. 96).

I believe that the vital technique we therapists need to master has to do with learning to re-cognize, to re-present to ourselves those moments when we inevitably become uninvolved and to reflect on how we can be and what we can do after that. And it is this technique, in the face of relational (k)nots, with which I concern myself here.[2] How do we allow ourselves, or gain the ability, to recognize and remain open to the actual lived pain or perturbation experienced in the therapy relationship when we come up against the sly repetitious negations that inevitably rub us the wrong way? How do we not ignore, patronize, pathologize, or move away from the person who is not saying that he considers us no better than a whore? How do we position ourselves to bear the possibility of feeling ambushed or tied up in knots and still sustain a process of involvement that both protects and promotes the analytic task?

How do we distinguish, in such untenable or dangerous moments, between moving away (toward negating or dissociating) and stepping back (toward perspective taking and reflective functioning)? Before attempting to illustrate, through a clinical vignette, the creative possibilities inherent in recognizing and releasing the relational (k)nots that inevitably crimp the treatment situation, I want to lay some groundwork by taking into brief account the role of reflective functioning in communication and development.

Making Room for Self and Other: A Two-Person Process with Involvement

In the title of a commentary on the work of Fonagy and his colleagues, Susan Coates (1998) succinctly operationalizes Russell's (1996) notion of "process with involvement," a process that has come to be defined as the capacity for reflective functioning. Coates (1998) calls it "Having a Mind of One's Own and Holding the Other in Mind." She writes:

> One of Fonagy's specific contributions has been to take a look at the microprocesses involved in the intergenerational transfer of secure and insecure attachment from one generation to the next. What he has found to be particularly relevant from a clinical standpoint is a component of parental sensitivity . . . which goes beyond affection, concern, and affect attunement and involves *the capacity to hold in mind the mental state of the other* (Fonagy et al., 1991). (p. 130, emphasis added)

In the words of Fonagy and Target (1998):

> It is assumed that the parent who cannot think about the child's particular experience of himself deprives him of a core of self-structure that he needs to build a viable sense of himself. We suggest that developmental personality disturbances arise first from the child's failure to find the image of his mind, his experience of himself as a thinker of thoughts, believer of ideas, feeler of emotions, in the mind of the caregiver. (p. 93)

Accordingly, these authors' research findings show that patients (in this case children) with complex developmental issues derive no benefit from "insight" or from treatment less intensive than twice weekly. The therapeutic action is centered in the unfolding patient-therapist relationship and its fostering of the capacity for reflective functioning. As Russell (2006a) puts it, "It is the actual successful containment in a relationship, with the therapist, that is the *agency* by which the capacity to contain is structuralized within" (p. 17). We can consider this as a kind of repetitioning of those crimps in development where the sense of self has dropped out. In ordinary development:

> The experience of containment involves the presence of another being who not only reflects the infant's internal state but represents it as a manageable image, as something that is bearable and can be understood. *The perception of the self in the mind of the other becomes the representation of the child's experience, the representation of the representational world.* (pp. 93–94, emphasis added)

That is, an affective-cognitive structure is formed within a two-person process.

What might the experience of noncontainment and nonrecognition mean for the daughter, the social psychologist, in our first vignette? Are we not impressed with how, in her conversation with Mother, her affect appears direct and intact? But how, in other moments of vulnerability, is she able to process her thoughts and feelings? What makes her still pursue her mother? What kind of relationship will she make with her own children? We can well imagine why this young woman became a social psychologist, and we can hope for the new meanings she may ultimately make of her work, her ability to nurture, and her capacity for attachment. Will we see her in our consulting rooms? Will our efforts to make a genuine attachment with her be crimped by avoidance, control, and (k)notted desire? What responses will these (k)nots evoke in us? What are the chances that we will remain involved, maintaining a mind of our own while holding this other in mind?

Introducing Simon

A Closer Look at Relational (K)nots and Potential Ways to Deal with Them

Simon B is a senior executive in a major advertising firm. Attributing much of his success to sharply honed communication skills, Simon is equally articulate about the ways in which he regards his mother, whom he has variously described as "unfulfilled," "needy," "intrusive," "not listening," "dependent on me," and "very insecure." On this day, he enters my office with an amused and conspiratorial smile that I do not recognize just then as a cover-up for unnamable affects. Having visited his mother on her birthday the previous week, he flips me a thank-you note that he wants me to read. Then he takes it back so that he can "perform" the message for me. He wants to know if I would like to try and figure out why this "nice letter" leaves him so disgusted and amused.

The letter begins with "Simon" (not the usual "Simon dear") and moves directly to the heart of the matter:

> Trying to connect up with you may delay this message, so I decided to put it on a note. As always it was great to be with you and Joanne and have you share dinner with me. It always seems so hectic. But I hope you enjoy coming as much as I love having you. Thank you so much for the beautiful gold bracelet. I love it and will wear it with pride.

And then with a flourish of the paper, Simon recites its closing sentiment:

> Gosh, each year the gift gets better. I can hardly wait till my next birthday.

At this moment in our session, Simon throws up his hands and laughs. I forget what I know about Simon—the ways in which he puts off returning his mother's phone calls, visits her in hit-and-run fashion, dragging along his reluctant wife. I forget how Simon's "superior" sort of distancing enacts his hatred of the many ways in which his mother's intrusive and narrow-minded neediness dictated his behavior in the past. I forget how difficult it is to join with Simon in a way that might lead us to a more intimate arena of experiencing. I forget the omnipresent promise of that potential between us and simply laugh along with him. And then I am aware of feeling sleepy, and I begin to think about other things as Simon goes on talking.

For reasons that I hope will soon become clear, I pause here once more to elaborate in more detail an etiology for my concept of relational (k)nots and outline some possibilities that might help to unravel them.

What could occur, developmentally, that would crimp the query "Is this me, or is this you?" Coates (1998) reiterates that the child who cannot find his mind in the mind of his mother "is left without an awareness" that he has a mind of his own . . . "without a personalized, authentic and vitalized sense of self." The space where the experience of "me" has been dropped out is now jammed by "parental preoccupations that are experienced as alien unmetabolized introjects, leaving the child without a sense of himself as a person in his own right" (p. 124). Hence the query, "Is this me, or is this you?" Coates explains:

A child whose reflective functioning has remained underdeveloped and compromised by the parent's preoccupations and defenses will be prone not only to breakdowns in functioning involving issues like separation, autonomy, and self-regulation, or the management of aggression, but also to breakdowns around those particular affect-event experiences where the parents' capacity to hold the baby in mind is profoundly compromised. (pp. 124–125)

I have already suggested that in severe pathology the (k)not may be seen as a preverbal tangle or strangle of agency so that when language forms, it forms around a crimp that has eclipsed the space reserved for a self's reflective functioning. But all of us have breakdowns around particular affect/event experiences where we "lose it" so to speak; all of us preserve, unwittingly, antiquated habits of mind that no longer functionally serve our purposes. ("Is this now, or was it then?") Furthermore, the presence in communication of another person's persistent (k)notting often evokes a (k)notting of our own. Relational (k)nots can be highly contagious.

Regardless of content, the (k)not has common characteristics and consequences. Here is how we may learn to recognize them:

1. The (k)not collapses potential space and paradox (see S. Pizer, 1998).
2. The (k)not is nonnegotiable.
3. The (k)not challenges/stunts affective development.
4. The (k)not is a negation of ownership of affect, wish, belief, intention.
5. The (k)not provides a kind of "grief insurance" that protects itself from the awareness of the pain of memory.
6. The (k)not is a device that dismantles/disassembles involvement.
7. And, therefore, (k)nots are repeatedly installed for the purpose of preserving attachments that are felt to be necessary for survival.

Before moving on with the case illustration, I want to generalize briefly about possible "techniques" that may encourage the releasing of relational (k)nots.

To begin with, of course, there is no fixed "technique."

What has to happen—and it does not necessarily happen first—is to recognize the existence of (k)nots. Discomfort with the way one finds oneself behaving or responding may signal a (k)not: a sense that the dialogue is repeatedly nonnegotiable or crimped, a sense of retreat from involvement.

The second necessary recognition by the analyst is that words seeking to explain the patient to himself will simply not suffice. There has to be a statement about how the two participants are and are not involving one another—about *the process* of what seems to be going on between them—rather than attempts to clarify a particular content.

The third recognition relates to the necessity for risk. The therapist/analyst (*or* the person in the patient's place) must offer something new, something that speaks to how his or her separate mind works—how he or she is thinking about what is going on, or an association he or she has. The disclosure here is greater than its words—it is an action, a jolt to the consciousness of both parties that may catapult the participants out of the familiar habits of the past. A disclosure here is best characterized as action, often a surprise to both participants, that may serve as a kind of counterweight to the original actions that occurred developmentally before the participants were armed with words.

Simon and Me

Simon had been coming to see me since the early 1980s. Direct and straightforward from the outset, he would usually tell me when our discourse threatened the approach of something he was not ready to pursue. Or I thought he did. He seemed so scrupulous, even in the tiniest detail, pausing to inform me each time he invented a name for somebody whose name he said he would rather not reveal. A deeply private man himself, he was particularly protective of other people's boundaries. I guess I felt so drawn to Simon—his integrity, his intelligence, his wry wit, his sweet demeanor—that I did not heed brief counterinstances of mood or pay attention to the moments when my mind would wander or my eyes would want to close. After certain periods of work together, Simon would smile appreciatively, announcing that he was in a better place than he had been before and that it was time to get on with his life. He certainly hoped that his departure would not be taken as a failure of accomplishment on my part. Demurring, I would graciously accede to his construction of events. Allowing a few weeks for closure, and with no inquiry from me, Simon would shake my hand and gratefully depart.

In our most recent engagement, however, I could immediately sense that Simon's return brought something new; something, I did not know what, had opened up for him. I experienced this new state, ironically, because of the depth and range of what he allowed me to see of the pain that now would play across his face. As for myself, I felt vitalized and alert.

This time he began our session by asking how I was. What had happened to me since he saw me last? Had I read any interesting books lately? Taking silent note that I was not put off by this particular mode of interview, I answered his questions.

"I get the sense," I said, "that you need to hear from me specifically as a way of reminding yourself who you may be talking to. Could that be so?"

Somewhat taken aback by my explicit formulation, Simon paused, then nodded.

"Somebody outside yourself," I went on. "A safe other. Maybe you need to know if you can trust me to hear whatever it is you might want to say ... and then speak to it from where I sit."

"Yes," was his immediate response. He took a breath. "I want to blame you for something that happened when I first came in to see you. I want to blame you for not stopping me from marrying Joanne."

Ruefully, I smiled.

Simon smiled back. "Only kidding," he said.

In the ensuing silence, I think we both experienced an awareness that he both was and was not kidding. His so-called joke allowed me to recognize—after more than a decade of sitting with him—how much (his need for privacy notwithstanding) I had allowed to remain unspoken between us and how I had acquiesced to innuendo without protest or inquiry. I understood this only now, in the face of the inexplicable change occurring between us. Simon was not holding me off in quite the same way anymore. I could actually see it happening in real time. I had a sense of his explicitly carving a space around himself, a sort of moat across which he could talk and safely maintain his position while getting to me.

"After all your training," he quipped, "can't we figure out something a little more original than the 'Mother is the Root of all My Problems' thing?"

Dumbfounded, I could think of no way to answer.

"It is true though," Simon went on, "they both get on me for not showing up. But every time I do, they're occupied! Yesterday, Joanne begged me to cancel my meeting and come home early because she wasn't feeling well. And guess what? I dropped everything, flew home, and when I got there with dinner, there was a note on the table. She went to the movies. *She went to the movies!*" Simon laughed. (In retrospect, I noticed that for once I did not automatically laugh along with him.)

Over the next months, Simon enumerated, in growing detail, incidents in which he had felt mistreated by Joanne. This was new for Simon. As he became less protective of me, and then of Joanne, and then of himself, I could palpably experience a diminishment of shame, both his shame and mine, which repeatedly seemed to take the form of silence and deferring to the will of another whom I perceived to be more powerful. Nevertheless, Simon, while clearly asking for "help," seemed to want to put a stop to my new-found freedom. As I became increasingly perturbed by the abusive nature of the scenarios that Simon would describe—incidents that, I inferred, both he and Joanne colluded in rapidly denying—as I questioned their relationship, Simon silenced me either by insisting that I tell him what to do or by upping the ante.

"So, what do you think about divorce?" he would say.

"A nightmare worse than death," would be my reply. "A last resort. But can't we try to figure out how you are *feeling* first, before we get to that extreme? Can't we take a look at how and why you are contributing to this going on the way it is?"

"So, what should I do?"

"Simon, you *know* I can't tell you what to do," I would sigh. "I can help you look at what's going on, I think, so you can figure that out for yourself."

Gradually, we began to make sense not only of the historical roots of his relationship with Joanne, but also of how he perpetuated the unspoken standoff that encapsulated their explosive scenes—meeting misrecognition with evasion, neediness with disdain, demands for more attention with a cool, deflecting cordiality.

"But even so," Simon insisted, "at some level, I really love Joanne. I feel so sad for her, that she has to behave like she does, so outrageous. I really can't bear the thought of leaving her."

We talked about the present and the past, the possible meaning that he made of love and its relationship to intense pain and such anxiety over any kind of leaving. "I know that between me and my parents it's over and done. They can't get to me anymore. I've made my peace with that. But Joanne, it isn't fair to her. She has nothing."

"Nothing?" I asked. "She has your pity, and she has your 'putting up with her.' What do you think that does for her inside?"

"I don't know."

At the time, I did not realize the passion or intensity that was driving my last question. It did not register in consciousness that I had crossed a line with him, and therefore I did not recognize the bland retreat in Simon's "I don't know." So I pressed on. "Well, I guess we really can't know about her. But what about you?" (I was not aware at the time that it was precisely Simon's familiar, somewhat righteous, implacable stance that had fueled my fire.) "You've really drummed it into me, to both of us, how important it is for you to maintain the status quo, how separations really do make you anxious. Do you think that may have to do with your staying with Joanne so long?"

"I don't know."

Angered by what I experienced as his steady and persistent challenge to my attempts at inquiry, I slowed myself down and made my voice go soft. "Do you think, Simon, that it's fair to her for you to bring out the worst she has to offer?"

He sat silent.

"Well, do you think that you could find your way back to loving her?"

"Don't know."

"Do you want to?"

"Want to what?"

"Love her. Try to love her"

"Sounds good."

"What do you mean, exactly? Say more if you can."

"I mean it would be good if I could."

I experienced my anger rising; a shortness of breath that annoyed me. "Actually, I have to say, I would hate it Simon, the way she goes after you and then you both deny it. That kind of business makes me crazy."

"*I could never hate her*," Simon retorted—somewhere from up on the ceiling it seemed to me.

Wait, I never said that. Or did I? What did I say? I felt a little crazy and duly chastised, the old shame burning at my neck.

"Thing is," he sighed at last, "I can't make it work and I can't leave."

As I sat there, taking in his latest words, all the while trying to disengage from my own bewilderment, remorse, and ridiculous outrage, Simon came back at me with an intensity that I had not experienced from him before, an intensity delivered from a distance that I could not reach, an intensity that took me over somehow and left me feeling stupid.

"I'm not capable of making a relationship," he hissed. "From what you know of me you must agree. Even if there does happen to be something better out there, something real, someone in particular, somebody who really loves me, somebody I could grow with, somebody like . . . I couldn't do it."

Somebody like whom? I thought to myself. *Whom is he talking about?* "What makes you . . . me think I could be there for that person?" he continued. "What makes you think that after the hash I've made of all my important relationships that I can do better—even if I gave myself the chance? *You were there when I tried it with Joanne.* You know that I'm incapable of making a relationship. Say otherwise, and you would just be misleading me again. Right?"

Beneath his polished and remote exterior, I felt Simon's face directly in my face. "*Right?*"

For an instant I understood clearly. I did not need any more words to comprehend that this man was actually telling me that he had fallen in love with another woman, God forbid—maybe even for the first time in his life—and he did not know what to do except to question me about it, hold me responsible for some kind of "truth" about how it would come out, while simultaneously telling me how impossible the whole thing was.

"So tell me," Simon pushed, "tell me what you have to say."

Now a blur. I found myself sitting in front of Simon, thinking of all the times my father had grilled and tested me when I was young (Was this moment now or was it then?): name the original thirteen states; why do we need a Bill of Rights? I felt myself experiencing my father's ruthless cross-examination of my ideas, remembering how much I hated this man I loved so much, this German Jew who went back to night school, this Doctor of Jurisprudence who was forced to flee his country and go back to school all over again for a second law degree, this Hitler refugee who, in the face of my hatred, *insisted that he never hated anyone or anything.* I sat there remembering how often I went dumb in his presence, how I wanted to cry, and all the while dreaming up fantastic rescue scenarios that he might admire, brilliant acts of accomplishment that would knock his bloody socks off!

"I want to hear what you have to say," Simon insisted.

"You're going through a process," I replied.

"Look," he pressed me further, "I'm a big boy now," he said with his familiar wry, disdainful smile, "I know how to think for myself. I'm asking what you think."

Is this me, or is this you? Did I do this, or was it done to me? I thought of my father, who taught me more than anyone else has ever taught me to think for myself, and who simultaneously still continues to inhibit my ability to take the time to speak my mind. Thinking about that paradox somehow released my mind.

"I can't exactly say what I think," I said to Simon, "but I'm reminded of a story."

"Tell me," Simon urged.

"It's a story that a close client of my father's told me soon after my father died. I should say that my father was a proud family man, who passed on to me many of the inherited traditions that he valued. Some I keep; others I have tried to let go. Well, this client, who had been miserable in a marriage of more than twenty years, fell in love for the first time with another woman. He didn't know what to do. He told my father that he knew he should give this woman up. 'Why is that?' my dad inquired. 'Love aside,' the client said, 'a twenty-year marriage has a history that is surely worth preserving.'"

Apparently my father shook his head.

"I can't advise you what to do," he said. "All I know is: You preserve antiques, you build relationships."

Silence between me and Simon. Then: "So you're telling me to leave Joanne."

"No," I replied, breathing freely now, "not at all." I felt oddly calm, at rest. "You asked me what I was thinking, and I decided to tell you."

"I remembered a story about a way to think about the thing you need to think about. I was thinking about a way of thinking that might help you begin to make up your own mind."

Discussion

Here is what I believe was happening between Simon and me, and how the story of my father's story served to open up a reflective space by untying the double (k)not that crimped our dialogue. As I look back, I can see that Simon (unconsciously) sought for me to become involved enough in his dilemma to keep him *uninvolved*. The enactment went like this: while persistently soliciting my views, he would repeatedly cut me off whenever he sensed that the direction of our conversation was heading toward territory outside the range of his own embedded, unreflective, and (k)notted "understanding." My own reciprocal valence for (k)notting had led me to intensify efforts to please, or go along with, the person I allowed to hold me hostage by an oscillating combination of promise, mind teasing, and ultimate unreachableness.

For Simon and me, the back-and-forthing of our pursuit and retreat loosened an awareness of my own preserved parental transference—a (k)not that now opened up to a new experience of pain and grief and love, an unfolding that made possible the recollection of a story that I could now convey for Simon's use and, even though I could not fully know it at the time, his potential unfolding.

In the months that followed, Simon gradually altered his persistent (k)notting course of wanting me to give him what he did not want as a way of preserving a familiar and wordless mode of relating. Suddenly, and at last, he saw the sense to my recommendation (which he had up to now doggedly refused or deflected) to undertake a couple therapy with Joanne.[3] And as Simon and I, in parallel with the couple treatment, engaged in an increasingly open exploration of the experience and meanings of his "secret" love, our dialogue—it seems to me—provided a kind of scaffolding for the experience and meaning of building a relationship.

Conclusion

As I suggested earlier and have also written elsewhere (see B. Pizer, 1997),

> *I believe that there are moments in the clinical process when the patient indicates a need or ripeness to receive, for personal use, some elements from the analyst's subjectivity.* That is, the analyst deliberately exercises her clinical judgment that the patient seeks—whether implicitly or explicitly—a sample of how the analyst's separate mind works. (p. 466)

There are also times of great surprise when the dialogue between patient and analyst becomes so crimped that the analyst's awareness of her own associations leads her quite spontaneously to offer some "other-than-me substance" (see Winnicott, 1969) that may open a space that analytic "clarification," "interpretation," "inquiry," or analytic silence may not provide.

At the moment of remembering and then deciding to tell Simon my father's story, I could not yet fully grasp its meaning for myself, nor could I predict its particular relevance for our subsequent work. But I believe that the act of sharing it with Simon may have yielded what Susan Coates (1998) describes as "the small mis-meeting of minds" that the negotiation between therapist and patient requires "if the patient is to be authentically met" (p. 128).

In summary, I would like to emphasize the resonance between the two-part process (repetition and containment) that Russell (2006a) outlined and I have illustrated here and Coates's (1998) commentary on the clinical implications of contemporary mother-infant research. Coates (quoting from a personal communication with Peter Fonagy) describes the function of repetition and containment in the treatment situation by explaining how one must "permit," and even in some circumstances "encourage," the patient to "colonize one's mind and then recover" in order to be able to offer the patient a fresh perspective on their own mental functioning (p. 127). And, Coates elaborates, "In effect, by responding in a way that suggests a degree of freedom in relation to affect, the therapist is providing an intentional stance of [her] own that invites the patient to do the same" (p. 128).

Whereas a relational (k)not crimps mental structure, the restoration of relational dialogue reengages the building of mental structures, containers of memory, feeling, and desire. As Russell (1996) would say, *"Structure is the passage of process with involvement"* (p. 216; emphasis added). But here the final words belong to Simon. Ultimately able to grieve what he had never found in childhood and what he could not make possible in a life with Joanne, Simon has become able to acknowledge his current love, and the pain of experiencing his love. He tells me now, "I have stopped seeing myself in my parents' eyes. I think less and less about who I am not, and more of who I am."

Notes

1 This chapter was first presented in 1989 at the Paul L. Russell Psychotherapy Symposium, Boston, MA.
2 It is important that we remain mindful of how unexamined elements of training and technique can engender relational (k)nots. Consider the notions of "proper analysis" or "standard analytic technique." Here lies the canon that requires us to talk about "alterations" or "modifications" of approach. And once we have empowered ourselves to decide that a patient is "too demanding," too "unable," suffering from too much "deficit," and once we set our own behavior to a standard of "too therapeutic" or "insufficiently analytical," we have seriously curtailed the relationship with the person we are trying to talk to. We are engaged, rather, in an unspoken relationship that most certainly perpetuates a relational (k)not. Furthermore, such a (k)not extends beyond the dialogue in our consulting rooms. It is an attitude that contributes to a continuing construction of theory based less on recognition of the persons we sit with and more on adherence to a nonexistent "norm" and justifications for deviating from it. It reifies tradition at the expense of living people.
3 By this time, Joanne had entered into a therapy of her own, and I thought it best for *her* therapist to make the couple referral.

References

Coates, S. (1998). Having a mind of one's own and holding the other in mind. *Psychoanalytic Dialogues, 8*, 115–148.

Fonagy, P., & Target, M. (1998). Mentalization and the changing aims of child psychoanalysis. *Psychoanalytic Dialogues, 8*, 87–114.

Laing, R. D. (1970). *Knots.* New York, NY: Pantheon Books.

Pizer, S. (1992). The negotiation of paradox in the analytic process. *Psychoanalytic Dialogues, 2*, 215–240.

Pizer, B. (1997). When the analyst is ill: Dimensions of self-disclosure. *Psychoanalytic Quarterly, 66*, 450–469.

Pizer, S. (1998). *Building bridges: The negotiation of paradox in psychoanalysis.* Hillsdale, NJ: The Analytic Press.

Russell, P. L. (1996). Process with involvement. In L. Lifson (Ed.), *Understanding therapeutic action: Psychodynamic concepts of cure* (pp. 201–216). Hillsdale, NJ: The Analytic Press.

Russell, P. L. (2006a). The theory of the crunch. *Smith College Studies in Social Work, 76,* 9–21 (written in 1987).

Russell, P. L. (2006b). The role of loss in the repetition compulsion. *Smith College Studies in Social Work, 76,* 85–98 (written in 1988).

Weakland, J. H. (1960). The "double bind" hypothesis of schizophrenia and three party interaction. In D. D. Jackson (Ed.), *The etiology of schizophrenia* (pp. 373–388). New York: Basic Books.

Winnicott, D. W. (1990/1969). The use of an object and relating through identification. In *Playing and reality* (pp. 86–94). New York: Basic Books.

Chapter 4

Passion, Responsibility, and "Wild Geese"

Creating a Context for the Absence of Conscious Intentions[1]

Stephen Mitchell (2000), in differentiating role responsibilities in the mutual but asymmetrical relationship between analyst and patient, writes,

> It is the analysand's job, in some very important ways, to be irresponsible. That is, we ask analysands to surrender to their experience, to show up and discover what they find themselves feeling and thinking. We ask analysands to renounce all other conscious intents. As we all know, this is not easy to do. (p. 131)

It is in this context that I ask you to surrender to the experience of this chapter—to go along with me without dwelling too much on the content until we're done, and then we can look back to see what meaning may be found.

The Analyst's Context

Although I am not a poet, I am drawn to poetry. It feels as though it is my medium. I love to read poems, to experience myself as fed by them; and when overwhelmed by an emotion or bewildered by an experience of uncertainty about stirrings from within, I often find myself sitting down and writing what one might call a poem. Going in and coming out, the thing has a tone to it, a music that I discover before I know where and how my words are traveling. I seem to be carried along by the tone of a developing idea or image, and it is the tone that dictates the rhythm and shape of the written lines. The music stops or goes flat when I come to an end of what has just emerged for me, and I am either disappointed or surprised.

If I feel surprise and the surprise brings pleasure, I begin to work on honing the progression of thoughts. I should probably say that by pleasure

DOI: 10.4324/9781032666303-6

in surprise I am not referring to a happy understanding or satisfaction in the solution sense—the words and phrases may just as likely capture some yearning or irresolvable sadness that is unaccounted for—but there it is, I can see it, I have begun to meet it. Now I am ready to question the language and the shape that I have let it take. A kind of dialogue takes place between myself and the lines that have been set down. What exactly have I evoked? Are the meanings clear and open rather than thoughtlessly borrowed from some cliché to fill a space or make a rhyme? Do the phrases of feeling and image come together? Do they ring a bell . . . set off some resonance or universal experience that may even urge me to share what I have arrived at so suddenly yet knew all along? Under the right circumstances, I may even read what I have written to a friend. Similarly, when I discover a poet's work that sings to me in a particular way, I am eager to read it aloud to someone who I think will participate in the experience.

How do I relate poetry to clinical practice?[2] There are times when I choose to read a poem to a patient. These are times when it seems that a particular poem, more than an interpretation of my own, will best interrupt a familiar ritual or provide by its surprise an unexpected opening, a play space, a soothing, or a saying of something difficult to hear but not unbearably humiliating, because it is spoken without the actual speaker present in the room and is spoken in some metaphor that can first be dealt with in the darkness and protected privacy of a quiet listener's soul.[3]

Am I specifically suggesting that the reading of selected poems is a useful clinical technique? No. I want to advocate for the idea of an analyst's bringing a relationship to something *other* into the consulting room, some source of vital nourishment outside himself or herself and outside his or her particular analytic school or identity. I'm talking about a passionate interest—be it stargazing, Buddhism, jazz, or ancient history—some counterpoint to the intimate task at hand that, even if never explicitly mentioned, brings air, texture, and dimensionality into the enclosed space in which two people are engaged. Perhaps we could call that passionate interest, that context that the analyst brings, the nonanalytic third.[4] By nonanalytic third I mean some timeless, personally constructed other that accompanies the analyst before the arrival and after the departure of a patient—a passionate interest that may also serve in the consulting room as a kind of placeholder for the potential in potential space. And it is just such an enduring object that can be relied on during the ultimate and necessary ending of an intimate analytic partnership.

I imagine that gathering these ideas into a concept called the nonanalytic third may be experienced somehow as odd, a bit playful for such serious intent. Nevertheless, I take on the phrase as a way of jolting our unreflective tendency toward logic or linear thinking. I am suggesting a kind of pun through condensation—joining paradoxical ideas in a single concept. That is, how does one decide what is or is not analytic in the first place, and if whatever it is originates outside an analytic school or relationship, how then do we conceive of the thing in terms of a third? More about this later.

The Patient's Context
Articulating Conscious Intentions

As Mitchell (2000) writes,

Analysands start out trying to accomplish all sorts of other goals: getting "better" quickly, avoiding trouble, taking care of the analyst, and so on. So we work with them on articulating their conscious intentions and discovering what would make it safe enough *not* to pursue them. *We are trying to create a context in which the absence of conscious intentions will allow feelings to emerge, feelings like love and hate.* (p. 131; emphasis added)

Mitchell stresses here that the most "analytically interesting" (p. 131) intentions tend to be unconscious, or "unformulated" as Donnel B. Stern (1997) would say. So our job is to employ our own emergent feelings in trying to facilitate those conditions wherein the patient can open to unattended passions, with the goal of getting to know those feelings and the part they may be playing in making, breaking, or masking a life. In Mitchell's words, "We are trying to cultivate in the analysand a kind of analytically constructive irresponsibility" (p. 131).

For my patient Sam, the very notion of irresponsibility triggers trouble, unhappiness, and deep remorse. More than thirty years ago, in one of the confusing off-again cycles of a long-term, passionate, on-again, off-again college love affair, Sam was suddenly struck and then smitten by an elegant and popular new woman on campus. He was just finishing graduate school when she became pregnant with his child. The idea of keeping the baby seems not to have been considered much—least of all when I inquire[5] about it in the treatment. When I ask him how he felt about the abortion, he describes a brief moment in the hospital when his Amy was wheeled back from the operating room, her face as white as the sheet that covered her, white as a sheet with the stain of her blood on its edge. How did he feel? He fainted dead away. How did he feel? He tells me that a few days later, he proposed to her.

I see Sam first in a couples context. It is the early 1970s. Amy complains that Sam is critical and controlling, righteous, and disdainful. Sam, a tall, broad-shouldered man with a boyish air, does strike me as controlling. In contrast to Amy's bright, conversational ease, Sam appears more wary, more deliberate in his choice of words. "Amy falls apart over strong emotions," Sam explains, "and she is sexually passive. And I feel jealous that she concerns herself with everybody else's needs but mine." Amy counters with a detailed rationale of her own, and in my presence the two of them manage to transform angry disappointments into formal conversation. Such conversations continue week after week, until finally one day Sam breaks the intellectual standoff with an ardent plea for them to make a baby. When she agrees, they terminate the treatment.

In 1991, seventeen years after I first saw him, Sam shows up again, alone. He wants some insight into why he works so hard to "fill in" for others and yet receives so little in return. As for his marriage, he is happy to report a few significant changes: two beautiful children, Allison and Robin, and he and Amy have "great sex." But their day-to-day relationship remains the same—"cordial" at best—and he notes within him a somewhat frightening and unrequited hunger for hugs.

According to Sam, Amy is not totally truthful in certain areas of their conversation; furthermore, she has a particular way of overriding him when it comes to the kids. A detailed inquiry reveals, however, that he too has certain secrets from Amy, holds back with her, primarily around his fantasy life. Although he describes these fantasies as sexual, when ultimately he spins them out for me, I hear a yearning for intimate connection that must be paid for by prowess. Being a good guy and a responsible citizen becomes a predominant theme. In the weeks that follow, I have a sense of Sam's deep yearning for intimacy and passion and his fear of it as well. When I suggest that keeping his intense fantasy life to himself will surely not promote the intimacy he yearns for with his wife, he gives me two clear reasons for his silence. In the first place, Amy wants no part of his expressiveness. Instead of feeling empathy for his response, say, to an intrusion by a neighbor or to his mother's repeated interruptions, she considers him rude. Her focus is on everybody else's comfort. "Second," he says, "if I tell her something, I'll never know what happens to it, where she stores it, what she makes of it." Perhaps for emphasis, he reiterates, "Don't forget, Barbara, Amy wants me to lighten up." Looking over at the sturdy gangle of his body slouched hopelessly across my couch, I somehow want to laugh at the sadness of all of this. "Amy doesn't talk to me about intimate things," he says.

I will have one year to work with Sam before he disappears for another six. The more I think that I understand what's going on, the more I don't. For one thing, I cannot comprehend the depth of warmth that he evokes in me. I am more accustomed to an unwelcome clutch of tension and effort when interacting with a man like Sam who maintains such vigilant control over what goes in and what comes out. But somehow I sense that Sam wants me to know, to find the person he keeps hostage, to recognize the wordless struggle taking place within him despite his massive efforts to contain it. I sense a history of both love and pain.

Sam is the child of a brilliant, alcoholic, and socially awkward father who nevertheless impressed and married a powerful, gifted woman—a passionate, articulate, and much-admired woman (widowed now and living alone just half a mile away), who cared deeply for her only son and loved and tended to her husband, all the while sparing no one declarations of her sense of right and wrong and proper living.

As for Amy's legacy and her relationship with Sam, I suppose I could offer a few hypotheses about the projective identifications and negative cycles that paralyzed their marital relationship, but those would simply be ideas of little usefulness to Sam or Amy or the purpose of this chapter. Sam and I would have to experience together what it was that needed to be learned. For example, if it were just Amy who hampered his expressiveness, what, at the moment, was holding him back in our work? What would be the context that might facilitate the absence of conscious intentions and allow feelings to emerge?

"Sam," I ask, "how is it that when I say something related to your current thinking, when I wonder what you have invested in a marriage you continue to complain about, you do like you haven't heard me, and go on?"

"I hear every word."

"What happens to the words?" I inquire.

"I park them," he says.

"So much for spontaneity," I sigh. "Can we talk more about your desire for closeness?"

"I yearn for closeness, and I fear losing it. I don't deserve it."

Sam's rationale that he is undeserving at this moment gives me pause. I have heard much about his growing up as an only child in an environment that he remembers as rich in love and hugs. Today, although he finds it hard to believe, he has become more established and gratified by increasing recognition for his professional accomplishments and academic contributions in a field related to my own. Currently, the obstacles to greater creative freedom are the constant interruptions from colleagues coming into his office for chats. "What stops you from closing your door?" I want to know. "An unwillingness to advocate for myself," he replies. By this time, I have learned to recognize affect and its intensity by Sam's arcane turn of phrase. Just now I am reminded of Sam's description of those times in adolescence when his father's drinking and the fights between his parents escalated.

"She would station me in the room next to theirs."

"What for?"

"In case he would get violent with her, so I could intervene."

"Pardon me?"

"So I could intervene."

I sit there with the image of a fifteen-year-old kid stationed on the other side of the wall—listening. What would constitute a signal? I ask Sam what would happen if, for the sake of pursuing his own agenda, he were to close his door. "Everything out there would fly apart," he says. This was one more instance, it seemed to me, of his desire—or rather, inhibition of desire—locked behind the door of perceived responsibility.

In that first year that I saw Sam (from May through the first weeks of June), he parked my suggestions about coming twice a week. He thinks about it some in early June, after a business trip where he finds himself disturbingly enamored by a female colleague's complimentary attentiveness. "Liza," he lingers over her name. "I wonder if I'll ever meet up with her again." And he wonders why he's wondering such a thing, in the same breath that he wonders where to take our process, or where our process might take him twice a week. Go one step deeper? Actually, it is not so much the money that's at issue here, but the time. It's time to leave, for now. He hopes that Amy will enter a treatment of her own. He promises to check back with me a year from now and, true to his word, he does just that almost exactly twelve months later. He comes to report that he hadn't bargained for how much more comfortable he would feel inside himself, for the keener sense of his own power that he now has. His colleagues seem to recognize and appreciate his many efforts, and even though the relationship with Amy remains the same, he experiences himself as easier and more accepting. He can see his contribution to the lack of intimacy in the marriage. Indeed he had been harsh with Amy, unkind . . . with certain rigidities about doing things his way, or his mother's way. He wants very much to let that go. I hope for him and for Amy; I wish him my best. And he is off again.

Now, alone in my consulting room, I find myself thinking about love and hate, desire and anger, and the weird prohibiting grip of my concerns about intrusiveness. I feel left to puzzle over Sam's expressed urgent need for holding recognition and all the ways he won't get close enough to share the risk of having what he says he wants so badly. "How odd," I tell myself, "that I should make this connection too late to share it with Sam. But of course!" I marvel, experiencing something between a smile and a sigh, "Sam got what he came for." Unthreatened by my closeness, he received just the recognition that he needed—moments after the door closed behind him.

About courting surprise, Stern (1997) writes,

> However deeply we may feel what we experience, and however passionate our commitments may be, spontaneous thoughts, images, or feelings are unexpected. They seem to come to us; despite the fact that our formulations are our own, we feel like conduits; our articulations of unformulated experience are unbidden. . . . Patient and analyst work with perceptions routinely. Most significant perceptions of others—of ourselves, too—arise without conscious intention. They come from elsewhere, unbidden, as symptoms or dreams. *They are events that fall outside expectation*, though seldom startling and not infrequent. Often they are the outcome of many small and half-noticed perceptions, the accretion of which, if it is noted at all, is seen only in retrospect. (p. 236; emphasis added)

A Context for the Absence of Conscious Intentions

Like dreams and like those moments of relationship when one feels fully present and alive, good poetry provides the opportunity to encounter events that fall outside expectation. To illustrate, and because Sam deeply loves nature and the outdoors, here are some stanzas from Mary Oliver's (1986) "Morning Poem":

Every morning
the world
is created.
Under the orange

sticks of the sun
the heaped
ashes of the night
turn into leaves again

and fasten themselves to the high branches—
and the ponds appear
like black cloth
on which are painted islands

of summer lilies.
If it is your nature
to be happy
you will swim away along the soft trails

for hours, your imagination
alighting everywhere.
And if your spirit
carries within it

the thorn
that is heavier than lead—
if it's all you can do
to keep on trudging—

there is still
somewhere deep within you
a beast shouting that the earth
is exactly what it wanted—

(pp. 6–7)

And so on. A poem, in its reading or writing, trains the mind to be in the present, to drop or question familiar patterns of assumption; to free-associate, to construct, deconstruct, and then construct again.

Now think about what makes for an absence of conscious intentions in Sam's dreams that I present here. The first was recounted to me on May 30, 1991:

I'm in my parents' once bedroom
It's a guest room now
With Amy and Marge
(Marge is a long-time friend of Amy's—
I saw her breast once, more of it than I think she knew)
And I see behind the fireplace an ember-briquette type vision.
I'm concerned the house will go down.

I try to get Amy's attention—to get water.
Amy says, "Just a minute, Sam,
I'm talking to Marge."

Six years later, he related another dream:

In not our current house . . . the first one.
Sparks are coming out of the wall.
Nobody is doing anything.
I see a fire truck outside the window.
It isn't stopping at the house.
Amy and Robin aren't doing anything.
I can't get through on the phone. . .

"Nobody doing anything," I think to myself. First house: Sam's passionate and self-involved mother who owns the only way to do things right and will not hesitate to tell you so; and his father, crazed by alcohol to calm his mood swings. That leaves young Sam on the other side of the wall, stationed to "intervene." I say none of this out loud, struck dumb by the sudden and forbidden wish to hold this huge man and tell him, "You're a grown-up now, you *can* get through, you *can* advocate on your own behalf!" At the same time I feel ripping mad at this guy who passes me his "nobody-doing-anything" paralysis while pressuring me to hold the pain. How to bear it? I cannot yet find my way clear.

Mitchell (2000) writes,

> In my experience ... love and hate emerge on both sides of the intersubjective engagement of the analytic relationship, but they have their own distinct qualities, different from love and hate in other contexts, and different for the two participants in the analytic relationship. . . . The analysand is asked to love and hate with abandon . . . . "Let yourself experience all these feelings that you have always regarded as most dangerous, so we can understand them, sort them out, and make them less terrifying." (p. 133)

And then Mitchell poses the question,

> What makes it possible for the analysand to feel safe enough to love and hate with abandon? In earlier decades, we might have thought it was the analyst's neutrality, anonymity, and abstinence that inspired such confidence. But there is now a widespread appreciation of how dangerous it is to love and hate with abandon an other who is hiding and posturing noninvolvement. (p. 133)

(We may think here of the power struggle between Amy and Sam.) Mitchell continues,

> What makes it possible to love and hate with abandon is involvement with an other who has feelings in return, sometimes even love and hate, but who is working to employ the feelings on both sides of the relationship in the service of analytic work— constructive, insightful growth and development. (p. 133)

It takes Sam two months to decide with me that his frustration and despair have arrived at the point where an analysis is worth a try. He now describes a third dream:

> *I'm on the Cape*
> *building a structure*
> *where my old kindergarten was,*
> *but on the dunes.*
> *The architect says—this will never hold!*
> *I watch a big dune—first a grain of sand . . .*

Then pebbles . . . then huge rocks . . .
I call to Amy and Robin,
Run for safety! Run for your life!

Sam remarks, "In this dream, I see it coming. Do you know what I mean? I'm surprised and not surprised."

As Stern (1983) articulates,

> The psychoanalytic process and the creative process have certain commonalities. In both, the process is emergent, not predetermined. The outcome is unknowable, and a final outcome is unreachable. In both, an initial stage of receptivity is followed by inspiration, then by application of directed, ordered thinking. In both, constructions appear, are honed, and then themselves become springboards for the next generation of constructions. (p. 95)

Sam and I, in our mutual but asymmetrical roles, seek a solid-enough context in which we may experience the absence of conscious intentions, precisely to uncover and hone the feelings we discover, for the building of a structure that will hold and then transform. Happily, my nonanalytic third prepares me for this task. For me, and at times for my patient and me, a poem serves as a container, an interpretative and creatively ambiguous opening for evocative experience that one or both of us can pick up and play with at will. A poem allows the possibility of recognition without pinning it down.

"Wild Geese"

Sam's face is bright from the out-of-doors when he comes in. "Walked over today," he informs me from the couch. He loves the briskness of air, and the telling to me of how he observes the seasons' changing—exactly where the sun sits in the sky, the color of the river. "No dreams," he says, and then, "The usual Amy story . . . she comes back with both girls an hour and a half later than she said she would. After supper, Robin is up doing her homework and it's time to take Alli back to the dorm. Amy says she's tired. So I say I'll go, but *she* goes, and she stays on and visits. I go up to bed with the outline that my new assistant, Julia, has written for my comments. At 11:45, Alli calls from the dorm to say that her mother is just leaving. So I turn off my light."

Sam continues, "This morning I wake up without a dream but I'm think-ing of Julia's body, and I have this image of a gushing fire hydrant." He gives me his Freudian interpretation. "Could well be," I say, "but you never know. Could be you're trying to put out a fire. Could be that you feel critical again, and angry because you think Amy is more interested in her daugh-ter than in you. Could be that you're trying to flush away or flush out the thought that Amy doesn't love you anymore, because you're so bad; so ... undeserving." Sam lets loose a disdainful grunt. I can tell that I will lose him momentarily. "Sam," I hear myself insisting, "a fire hydrant can be some-thing more than just a penis."

"What do you mean, '*just*?'" he jokes.

I am rifling through the papers and books piled on the table beside my chair. "I'd like to read you a poem, Sam," I say, "if it's okay with you."

"Okay, sure."

"It's by a woman named Mary Oliver. It's called 'Wild Geese.'"

"Okay."

> You do not have to be good.
> You do not have to walk on your knees
> for a hundred miles through the desert, repenting.
> You only have to let the soft animal of your body love what it loves.
> Tell me about despair, yours, and I will tell you mine.
> Meanwhile the world goes on.
> Meanwhile the sun and the clear pebbles of the rain
> are moving across the landscapes,
> over the prairies and the deep trees,
> the mountains and the rivers.
> Meanwhile the wild geese, high in the clean blue air,
> Are heading home again.
> Whoever you are, no matter how lonely,
> the world offers itself to your imagination,
> calls to you like the wild geese, harsh and exciting—
> over and over announcing your place
> in the family of things.

(Oliver, 1986, p. 14)

I do not know Sam's initial response to the poem, because he is silent for a long time. When he speaks, he talks about carefree high school days.

He talks about the passion and despair he experienced throughout the crazy on-again, off-again relationship with the woman he knew before Amy. He talks, as he tends to do these days when feeling vulnerable, about his fantasies—particularly about his fantasy of Liza. He saw her once again, by accident, in Paris last year. Things between him and Amy reached an all-time low. Sam felt lost in their power struggles over what was best for the children; it was three against one, he felt. Amy became so angry and heartbroken by his sulk and retreat from Alli that she fed him his own medicine in the one place where some form of communication was possible—bed. They hadn't made love for months. That was the event that brought Sam back to see me—his experience of being cut off by Amy, coupled with the fear and terrifying wish that he felt, away from home, when he bumped into Liza in Saint-Germain. They spent a long evening over dinner and wine, talking and talking. Then Liza went back to her fiancé, and Sam, weeping in a way he never (and always) had known, returned to his small hotel. He lay awake until the sun came up, fantasizing another life entirely. Had he totally lost his mind?

The day after he heard "Wild Geese," Sam came in with a question. "Do you have a supervisor?" he asked. "Why?" I queried, hoping to cover the feeling of a sudden blow to the stomach. "Because," he said to me, "I'm very worried that if I tell you how upset I was after hearing that poem, you'll retreat and I don't want you to." Throughout this session, Sam talks about how the poem "shook him up." What does this mean? He finds himself "tearing up" in the car, "just tearing up over nothing in particular." Now I remember his slip from the day before. He is talking about the image of the fire hydrant. He means to say that it is "exploding" with water, but it comes out "exposing." I think again about his question: "Do you have a supervisor?"

Between the two of us, who actually had been exposed? What elicited my frightful shame? Was it Sam's rubbing my face in outrageous analytic behavior? Was it the shocking freedom or power I heard in his tone? Or all of the above? In retrospect, I believe it was the first time I experienced between us, in the room, the raw presence of anger, shame, freedom, and desire. "Do you have a supervisor?" Had I made a terrible mistake? Shamed him by surprise? Was Sam handing over his internal supervisor and asking me to handle it myself? Could we ever know the many meanings of his unparked response to my reading "Wild Geese" to him? Because my repeated probing never produced contradicting material from Sam, we must remain content with his insistent, and perhaps one-sided, view that he feared somebody would stop me from working with him in the way I did, that when he let me know how truly painful it felt to open up to feeling, I would turn "responsible." Or somebody else would "intervene."

Over the next months, we recognize that something has opened between us. We are both aware, also, that our poem is no more than a place marker, a way station shared along an uncharted course toward a destination that cannot be predicted until we get closer—if we ever do. And we can note together—between the seemingly endless tedium of days on days—small arrivals and crossings over dangerous terrain. So it goes. To illustrate: Sam, who has been invited to join Amy in her therapy sessions with Jean Pelham, had his first one over the weekend. "In the middle of our session with Jean Pelham," he says, "I was talking about my need for intimacy, and you can guess what happens next. Amy said, 'there you go again, criticizing me!' As if that was my intention! So Jean asked me if I *have* any intimate relationships. Legitimate question; she must already know the nature of Amy's relationships. I didn't want to tell her the number of friends I grew up with and still have, so I mentioned Paul and Richard from work; I didn't say Julia. Then I said, dangerously, that I have an intimate relationship with you. When we left Jean's, Amy didn't say a word. That was three days ago, and not a word about our session."

"Did you bring it up?" I ask.

"I was planning to," he says. "At 11:00 that night, she was cheerfully going about her business, and I said, 'Let's go to bed,' so we could talk without Robin overhearing us, and she said she'd be up in a minute. Well, you know what's next. The last time I looked at the clock it was midnight. I went to sleep, and that was that." After a silence, Sam continues, "If I were to vanish," he muses, "I wonder if she would live her life differently. Amy went back to work after that couple session. I went home, and I cooked us this great meal that was cold by the time she got there." And then, "You know what? It's Amy's way when there is work to be done at the office. Amy would rather not eat . . . would rather be hungry than think, 'There is something I could do for Sam and me.'"

"And you? How would you construct your astounding situation?"

Sam sighs, "I'd rather be lonely in my marriage than feel . . ." Sam pauses. "The word *responsible* came into my head." He shifts position on the couch. "I have an image of me in the sunshine . . . fresh air. I'm out of the house . . . feeling kind of . . . airy . . . as if the figure of myself is out of proportion . . . sort of . . . disintegrated patches of me on the left."

"What do you think is going on inside the house?" I ask.

"Well, I'll tell you. It's the image of the house I grew up in and was younger in . . . the yard is less overgrown. It's a point of view I never would have had . . . me as big as the house and—"

I hear myself interrupt him. "You did have to grow up pretty fast. It goes with being responsible." There is a long silence. "You can't fix it, Sam," I say. And the hour is at an end.

Passion and Responsibility and a Nonanalytic Third

Just as I believe that stories about people are never neat or complete, the ideas and themes that have unfolded thus far in this writing—also not complete—have a history and a future I cannot claim. We all must be aware that ideas become unique as they are discovered, lived, and used by the people who receive them (see Levenson, 1983; Stern, 1997). So one aspect of what I intend to be writing about is the dialectic of responsibility and guilt over freedom from responsibility—the sort of guilt worn like a raincoat over love and hate, anger and desire. Similarly, I want to address passion and martyrdom as a defense against that passion. And I'm not just talking about Sam. I'm also talking about the analyst's passion and about a nonanalytic third as an alternative to martyrdom. More needs to be written about the life and love and losses in a good treatment, from the analyst's side; about those creative sources that ground the analyst's need to give, or risk, and then let go when it's time to let go of relationship without such acts collapsing into selfless sacrifice. And more needs to be written *about the facilitating of unformulated experiential space for the patient's use and about how one learns when the time is right to move forward in a more clarifying way.*

Actually, this chapter is constructed in the hope of coming closer to reexperiencing—rather than merely weighing from some analytic distance—the unfolding case of Sam and me. I have attempted to convey a flavor of the ambiguity, imprecision, and uncertainty that may be entailed in striving for the absence of conscious intentions in the analytic relationship. At this particular juncture, I have no idea how Sam and Amy will come to terms with their marriage. But as you see, an answer to that question cannot fully satisfy our overall quandary. Impossible as it may be to dwell too long in the absence of "memory and desire" (Bion, 1967), how do we *know* when the time is right to move forward in a more consistently clarifying mode? How do we learn to feel our way toward making and taking more explicit points of view, thus narrowing the open field for the express purpose of arriving at that necessary, often arbitrary, clearing where analysand and analyst part company?

I don't think we can know ahead of time. As for Sam and me, I learned long after the fact when we were suddenly shunted into what we may one day call the middle phase of our work. And in this conclusion, I must give you some indication, even if ever so briefly, of how we found ourselves shocked into such a seemingly new place.

Both Mitchell (2000) and Stern (1997) concern themselves with delineating a context for the absence of conscious intentions so that unformulated experiences are free to emerge. In our case, Sam's and mine, I believe we had constructed the context of safety that Mitchell has referred to. Then, for us, the reading of a poem helped to create another contextual aspect stressed by Stern—an element on the other side of safety—the preservation of uncertainty, the making of a space between experience and expectation. I wonder now if I am stretching a point to suggest that we unwittingly had prepared ourselves to navigate a new, uniquely impinging, and certainly unexpected nonanalytic third, which we were ready and able to make use of but would never have wished for and could never have predicted.

In the beginning of September 2001, Sam has to interrupt our work for a business trip abroad. Given his current research into the intersubjective processes by which people construct meaning with each other, I had already suggested that he look at Stern's (1997) *Unformulated Experience*. Before he leaves, he tells me he is taking this book along with him—partly for his work and partly to keep our work alive.

On September 12, I receive a message from his office on my answering machine. "Professor B. has asked us to let you know his plane has been diverted to Paris, and he has to cancel until further notice. Also, he would appreciate it if you would check your e-mail."

Wednesday, September 12, 2001

Hi Barbara,
I feel a real need to be in touch with people I care about—and who care about me. Could you let me know if you'll be checking your e-mail?

I'd like to get down a few thoughts. One is how grateful I am for your warmth and wisdom.

Sam

Because e-mail is not my medium, I avoid giving out my e-mail address, and I certainly don't give it to patients. But Sam is resourceful.

Dear Sam,
Now that you ask, I will of course be checking my e-mail. I got the message from your secretary. She sounded very upset and anxious, as are many people around here. My current diagnosis of your state, Sam, is that whatever else is going on with you, your reality testing is intact. You know that I care about you.

Dear Barbara,
This is the same little hotel I stayed in when I was here three years ago and suddenly bumped into Liza on the street. What a life-altering experience. I'm half a block off Saint-Germain.
 When they took us off the airplane Tuesday, I knew I didn't want to stay at the airport—that this could be a long stay. So I took a cab to this area. . . . I needed the familiar and was also indulging in the past. I am often thinking about Liza, and I actually mustered the courage to call her from here and tell her where I was. I had a good talk with Amy, too, a bit later. . . . All kinds of trouble getting through, a matter of phone lines, but I could feel how that summoned up a lot of our past. Even so, I felt open and after much detail-talk, said that seeing the video of the second plane flying into the tower again and again has made me profoundly aware of unfinished business.
 I recalled a recent Jean session in which Amy said, quite fervently, that if we were to get anywhere, together or apart, we would have to forgive each other—and ourselves, she added. So I told her in complete honesty that she owes me no apology and need ask for no forgiveness. If I get creamed, I wouldn't want her thinking—wrongly—that she did. And I truly feel that. I said that we may not be a good match. And maybe we need to recognize that and move apart, or recognize it and laugh it off. But I don't blame her. I really don't. And that actually feels very liberating for me.
 Lest you think I've gone completely soft, I can still be puzzled and angry about her behavior. On Tuesday 9/11 she got home from work at

6:30 or 7:00. Robin had been home for a couple of hours on her own and didn't know where in the world I was, quite literally. I just don't get why Amy's first impulse isn't to drop everything and be with her daughter. But if I can be critical of that, even self-righteous, I don't feel as if she somehow owes me something on account of that. Does that make any sense?

And let me associate to something else entirely. I just recalled my own disproportionate anger toward Bill Foster, the manager of the club who, I told you, has given my blind friend (and others) such a hard time. On the phone, Liza was saying that she just couldn't comprehend how someone could be so angry that they could destroy the lives of innocent people—and themselves in the process. She was speaking of the suicide pilots, of course. But I can understand it, sort of, at least, just knowing how powerful my own rage can be. And that rage lives someplace inside of me, notwithstanding the fact that I'm not feeling it now and seldom do, consciously.

My mind has been spinning about all such things and more while I've been here. Thinking about Liza and Amy, thinking about myself, trying with some success to be in the moment while walking from the Louvre up through the Tuileries toward the Champs-Elysées. There are times when I've been depressed and I've thought that I don't care that much about life, but that image of the plane has shocked that out of me in a way that nothing else ever has. "Want to hear my fantasy?" I can hear you say at this point (or more accurately, I wish I could hear you say that). That's not in the cards in this medium, but I do carry that image with me, and it is comforting and warmly amusing, too.

Dear Sam,
My God, is it already three years ago—that hotel in Paris where your whole world flipped over? Re: your straw-man comment. I don't think you have gone "completely soft." Au contraire, I feel that you have been shocked—like you were shocked three years ago when you ran into Liza in Paris, but this time you were shocked because the death part of the life-and-death experience came first, once again shocking you into a level of life in which you are more removed from what you know and feel, and simultaneously more sharply aware. Removed is definitely the wrong word; more at a distance from, say, your rage so that you can feel its power more acutely because you are not directly in it.

I agree that Amy doesn't owe you. The question is, do you owe Amy the something-or-other to tell her your bewilderment? How would your response be so different now? And do you know how you might express it in a way that doesn't intend high-minded blame? I wonder if the rage inside you is more powerfully awful than your inhibition against it? Time to close this down for now, Sam. Take care. Let me know when you are coming home.

Barbara

Hello Barbara,
Thank you so much for your reply. It was all the more welcome, as yesterday I felt very disconnected and hungry for hugs. Much of my immediate need was probably set up by an e-mail from Amy earlier. (Whoops, where did forgiveness go?) She gave a quick account of travel information, then closed with "I'll try to e-mail again later, but this place is sprouting deadlines and new work like mad, so I'm not sure when." That was her one message of the day. I truly don't get it. She is very worried about me; I know that from when we talk on the phone, but that was her one message of the day. And she wasn't able to get home to Robin until 7:30.

I've been reading Unformulated Experience—*it's quite remarkable. Stern writes about "familiar chaos," which reminded me immediately of Amy. Two quotes on page 51 that struck me in particular: "a state of mind cultivated and perpetuated in the service of the conservative intention to observe, think, and feel only in well worn channels—in the service actually of the wish not to think." Then a bit later: "The masochist for example does not refuse to acknowledge a fact he already knows; rather, by interpreting and living his life in a way that allows fulfillment of a cherished self-characterization—that he is giving, selfless, and perhaps victimized—he manages not to spell out the observations he could make if he were willing to tell a different story and consider alternative interpretations of his own place in it."*

Those passages struck a chord. To me that fits Amy to a T. And I am also trying to turn those very words—"giving, selfless, and perhaps victimized"—on myself and imagine a different story, and a different place in it. But it's so hard for me to do that right now—feeling the anxiety of not being home while not knowing what sort of home I'm coming home to. There are times when I'm okay. This morning at Air France I was in a band of expatriates, strangers in the conventional sense but people

who really have an inkling about what others are feeling and the result-
ing urge to connect with one another. While waiting for my number to
be called, I overheard a woman being short with her husband, more
desperate than angry, when the counter attendant told them that their
flight may be canceled. I spoke to them as they were leaving—none of
us has any particular place to go—and we quickly cut to the emotional
chase. She said she was crying all day yesterday, but that nobody else
is crying. I said, my own eyes welling up, that maybe she just hadn't
seen others' tears. I'm sorry if this is hard to read from afar, but it
was actually a good moment, something that allowed me to express my
humanity. It was such a welcome contrast to what I had experienced
the day before. We didn't have to say anything else; there was perfect
understanding.

Not without reason, though, is all this called terrorism. It really
works. I can see the shadows sweep over me from time to time. I try to
be mindful, but the thoughts often come rushing back. This little room is
confining and the constant CNN may not be a good thing, but sitting and
writing makes me feel better, particularly writing to you, as someone
who truly cares to listen. Thank you so much for being there. Give that
husband of yours an enormous hug.

Dear Sam,
I'm so glad you have Stern with you—so much your kind of guy in a time
when you have the time to think and feel deeply, even if alone. Of course
you are anxious about not being home. But I sense that you are begin-
ning to get a fuller sense of what you are coming home to in the way of
your immediate personal world— yours, Amy's, yours and Amy's. As
for the larger world, it is startling to try to comprehend the things we
have kept unformulated for so long. And now the unthought known keeps
blowing up in our faces, and we have no choice but to deal with it—each
of us in our own idiosyncratic way. You are not hard to read, Sam—your
experience, I mean, your moment of tears. Gadamer, as you must have
read in Stern, has that great expression for the perfect understanding
you describe—a fusion of horizons (Stern, 1997; emphasis added). This
is what connection is about, right?

I will send you a hug now, in the one way that I can. Listen as I read you
this poem. It is by Czeslaw Milosz (2001) and it's called "Incantation."
(You pronounce him Ches-wah Mee-wash.)

Dear Barbara,

I loved the poem—and the way that you read it with soft, clear urgency.
I heard your every word. I'll head to the airport in several hours. I'd say
it's 50/50 that I'll be in Montreal late Saturday evening.

Sam

Mitchell (2000) writes,

> The potential spaces psychoanalysis makes possible—sometimes poten-
> tial spaces filled with romantic love—have a life span. They can be enor-
> mously analytically useful, but only for a while. Then they can become
> constricting. . . . Ultimately it falls to the analyst to make decisions about
> the constructive versus destructive implications of various affects in both
> participants in the analytic process, even though there is no way to make
> those judgments purely objectively. Part of the analyst's responsibility
> is to participate in and enjoy that love, while it seems facilitative of the
> analytic process, but not to enjoy that love so much that it becomes a
> vehicle for the analyst's own pleasure in a way that occludes his focus
> on the patient's well-being. (pp. 138–139)

And so the last words belong to the man whom I call Sam. We have named
him together, after he has given me permission to write this chapter.

November 3, 2001 Dream:

> *I dream of a cheerful baby. Three months old? I ask myself. No, maybe*
> *six, I refigure. I want the baby to be strong enough. I pick him up and*
> *can feel the strength in his back. His skin is baby soft and warm. He says*
> *"Daddy." I am doubly astounded: I have a son? He can talk? I ask if*
> *he knows that he is precocious. Even if he doesn't know that word, he is*
> *very wise and comfortable with his wisdom. He says some other things,*
> *while being open and looking around. I ask his name (though I should*
> *know). It is Sam. It is strange that I have no idea who is his mother.*

Clinical Notes, July 25, 2003: "Naked and Potent"

An earlier version of this chapter ended here. Some readers of that version
have wondered what happened to our analytic work when Sam came home
from Paris. How did he look back on our e-mail correspondence? What
was its effect on the treatment? What conclusions, they asked me, do I draw

from these rather unconventional exchanges between us, and where do they fit in the overall frame of the work, as I perceive and present it? Some of those who asked me these questions also have said that they felt moved by the chapter without quite knowing why or have commented that they didn't know what to say about it after they finished reading it.

Could such an initial absence of speakable response be one purpose of the work as I have set it down? Perhaps, in this case, the medium is the message. I'm asking *us, as analysts*, to go through once more what we ask *our patients* to do. The suspending of preconceptions, the surrendering to process, can be like listening to a new poem or a beloved piece of music; it takes a while to come back from experiencing its tones and nuances before finding the words to formulate an articulate response or ask a question. Maybe such an exercise makes for new learning about ourselves and our patients.

But now, perhaps the time has come to elaborate in a more clarifying sequence some of the ideas I came in with, and came to, in my work with Sam. First, I am not alone in the conviction that no one—maybe least of all the reporting analyst—can ever really presume to *know* the specific causes or outcomes of particular therapeutic interventions or events (see Davies, 1999, pp. 195–196). Growth, changes, and transformations do not occur in linear fashion. For instance, I remember working many years ago with a kind and creative psychiatrist who was sexually potent in a happy marriage and who entered treatment with an intention to undo a block that prevented orgasm when he masturbated. To my knowledge, this had not been accomplished by the time he terminated his analysis, but for reasons unknown to both of us, he stopped biting his nails.

For patient as well as analyst, the effort to be with and listen openly to another is a tall order. There really is, in practice, no such thing as a total absence of conscious intentions. But, as analysts, we strive to come as close to that absence as we can within the givens of our asymmetrical roles, and we encourage our patients to do likewise. As analysts in our consulting rooms, we try to apprehend something of the moving landscape within and between each of us as the interaction proceeds before we attempt to define a provisional course.

One portion of the internal landscape that I come in with contains a love of poetry, and however it may contribute to experiencing with patients, there is also a way in which it feels quite separate from, or independent of, psychoanalytic work. A poem sustains me, keeps me company outside the clinical enterprise; and in that sense I consider it nonanalytic. At the same time, of course, poetry trains my mind toward openness and acceptance of surprise.

Clearly, my bringing the potential of poetry into analytic discourse with Sam was of use to us. Early on in our work together, we learned that doors—both open and closed—were of particular significance. As a young man, Sam experienced untenable rage behind a closed door. Face-to-face with an intrusive, penetrating maternal presence, Sam built himself an internal firewall that equipped him to create the appearance of open access while maintaining vigilant control over what came in and what went out. If things got really bad, he could withdraw with no one knowing it, and when they got worse, he could always disappear . . . however, not without cost to him of a more genuine spontaneity and the intimacy he claimed to yearn for most. So I believe that my offering the potential of poetry into analytic discourse allowed him to experience an other voice between us—indirect and multimodal, the primitive and essential prosody of a communicating process whose particular meanings he could find on his own if he chose to. That experience, I believe, contained the possibility of transforming in him a historical and calcified habit of shutting down at the threat of impending intrusiveness and shock, thereby permitting me, at times, to overcome my own historical and transferential tendency to feel outrageous in my efforts to speak my mind or, as Sam might say, to "advocate for myself." The "Wild Geese" experience, I would like to believe, became a prosodic process that provided us a kind of unwitting procedural preparation (or thirdness) for dealing creatively with the reality of an unanticipated other. We somehow managed to speak, to even sing to one another from a great distance, during the shared terror of 9/11.

Finally, bearing in mind that our work is still in process, or progress, and remembering that our acknowledged mutual caring has a limited life span in the analytic endeavor, I now relay verbatim my notes from the first hour of Sam's return to the office after coming home from Paris.

I sit down to write immediately after he leaves, entitling the session in red—"*Naked and Potent*." I can't remember how we began exactly; Sam just stood in front of me. I concentrated very hard on staying in contact and not hugging him. I felt glad to see him. He smiled. He gets on the couch, facing me, and recounts the story of his coming home: about discovering his old friend Linda Mason on the very same plane, and the "next nexus" of making a new friend who happened to sit beside him. Then he talks about landing in Montreal, calling Amy, and getting the answering machine. Telling this, Sam bursts into tears.

The next night—Sunday night—he describes asking Amy to come to bed. She tells him she will, after she does something or other. Twenty minutes later, he hears the dishes clinking downstairs—he's in a rage. He goes upstairs to his home office to check his e-mail, to see if there's a reply from Liza—nothing there—goes back down. Amy comes to bed. He moves from his usual side of the bed over to the left, to Amy's place. Amy questions this. He says he wants to be in a different position. They . . . he doesn't know what to call it . . . have long foreplay. He is feeling "very potent," he says to me, "ending in intercourse. It's not Amy," he continues, "it's not rape . . . but a sense of feeling powerful. Naked and potent," he says, as if surprising himself, "naked and potent at the same time."

I am silent. I associate to the fire hydrant . . . feeling exposed, and then I associate to "naked and potent at the same time" and his e-mail about his powerful rage. Creative use of his shame and power, I wonder? Image of Sam in a new position . . . coming back . . . into himself? But somewhere earlier in the session—I almost forgot—and I don't know precisely where in the sequence of things, Sam tells me how meaningful, helpful, "healing" it was for him, anxious in Paris, to hear from me (a rare direct acknowledgment). And how *he heard the poem in my voice!* I tell him, easily, that our work is hard work, but love is no effort. He smiles broadly and says, "and I love you. And it feels good to say." Sam tells me that he saw an episode of *The Sopranos* and the part where Tony declares his love to Dr. Melfi. He tells me that Dr. Melfi saw this as progress. And later in the show, Tony puts his arms around his wife, Carmella.

At the end of the session, I acknowledge our perhaps awkward moment when we began today at the door; perhaps he was standing for a hug . . . my awareness of that possibility . . . my wish to not reject him, along with a clear resolve that this was not the time for me to give him a hug. Sam laughs as he moves to open the door. "But you already did." He pauses. "And in Paris, the concrete hug. Anything you would give me now would be less than that. And we would only have to let go."

So that is the narrative of Sam's return from Paris. I would wish to hold those moments longer, but I am also aware that hanging on too long is liable to mislead us. When we consider Mitchell's question (2000)— "What makes it possible for the analysand to feel safe enough to love and hate with abandon?" (p. 133—we have to recognize that Sam and I have not yet fully grappled with the second half of what still is left to do if we can. Direct expressions of anger, for Sam as well as for me, will not come easily between us. I recall again, in this present context, how I once asked Sam why he persisted in keeping his door open to invasive colleagues and how he answered that he was unable to advocate for himself. It has taken me so long to re-cognize that, given his early history and despite external appearances, he knows all too well how to keep his internal fire door shut tight against intrusion, against exposure. Sam still parks some of my comments, and when I experience myself in a fusion of horizons with him, he is prone to imagining a sort of personal merger—that either I hold his agenda or I impose one of my own. At these times, I still feel powerless and prone to retreat in shame. I hope we can learn more about this unhelpful interaction together. Together, I hope we can figure out how we may both be able to move forward in a more clarifying way. I hope that Sam won't disappear, so we can try to accomplish this valuable piece of work before he leaves.

And that takes me back to the nonanalytic third and my initial question. How do I relate poetry to clinical practice? Is the reading of selected poems a useful clinical technique? No. But it is not unusual that the analyst's nonanalytic third is transformed in the consulting room and does indeed serve the intimate partnership as an analytic third. Poetry has served Sam and me for a good while in our analytic endeavor, because it is compelling yet indirect and can be picked up, related to, played with, or put down at will. Yet, like love and hate experienced in the work between us, it too has a life span. And I must emphasize once more the salient and defining feature of a nonanalytic third. What makes it nonanalytic is its one-person feature. Not simply an other that brings life into the consulting room, the nonanalytic third originates as the analyst's personal other that she has chosen for her own, that accompanies her before the arrival and after the departure of a patient. And it is just such an enduring object that can be relied on during the ultimate and necessary ending of an intimate analytic partnership.

Notes

1 I am grateful to Sue Elkind, June Margolin, Andrea Massar, Suzi Naiburg, and Stuart Pizer for their incisive and useful comments on a draft of this chapter, a shorter version of which was presented at the Inaugural Conference, the International Association for Relational Psychoanalysis and Psychotherapy, "Relational Analysts at Work: Sense & Sensibility," January 19, 2002, New York. I am also indebted to Sam (the patient whose case I discuss), and to Donnel Stern, Virginia Goldner, and Spyros Orfanos.

2 See Hoffman (1998): "It's time, perhaps, in general, for us to accept the responsibility to be artful and poetic in our work as analysts, since, in fact, we are always creating relational experiences, not merely studying them" (p. 802).

3 Davies (1998) in response to Hoffman: "[A] poem captures experience, holds it in evocative and linguistic forms, potentiates rather than forecloses the mutual negotiation of meaning contained within its words, and promotes perspectival awareness of multiple meanings, nuances, and potential interpretations" (p. 820).

4 Thanks to Stuart Pizer, who (after listening to me struggle with the formulation of this concept) thought up the term *the nonanalytic third* and suggested that I work it out from there.

5 I introduce the present tense here in the clinical narrative even though I am describing events that occurred years ago. I will at times in this chapter shift my stylistic use of narrative tense from past to present in an attempt to locate the reader more fully in the "present" moment of each clinical event no matter when it occurred. The implicit nonlinearity of time is intentional and consistent with my wish to invite the reader (as Mitchell asks analysands) to surrender to experience, to approach a state of "absence of conscious intentions."

References

Bion, W. (1967). Notes on memory and desire. *The Psychoanalytic Forum*, *2*, 272–273, 279–280.

Davies, J. M. (1998). Thoughts on the nature of desires: The ambiguous, the transitional, and the poetic: Reply to commentaries. *Psychoanalytic Dialogues*, *8*, 805–882.

Davies, J. M. (1999). Getting cold feet, defining "safe-enough" borders: Dissociation, multiplicity, and integration in the analyst's experience. *Psychoanalytic Quarterly*, *68*, 184–208.

Hoffman, I. Z. (1998). Poetic transformations of erotic experience: Commentary on paper by Jody Messler Davies. *Psychoanalytic Dialogues*, *8*, 791–804.

Levenson, E. A. (1983). *The ambiguity of change*. New York: Basic Books.

Milosz, C. (2001). *New and collected poems (1931–2001)*. New York: HarperCollins.

Mitchell, S. A. (2000). *Relationality: From attachment to intersubjectivity*. Hillsdale, NJ: The Analytic Press.

Oliver, M. (1986). *Dream work*. New York: Atlantic Monthly Press.

Stern, D. B. (1983). Unformulated experience: From familiar chaos to creative disorder. *Contemporary Psychoanalysis*, *19*, 71–99.

Stern, D. B. (1997). *Unformulated experience: From dissociation to imagination in psychoanalysis*. Hillsdale, NJ: The Analytic Press.

Chapter 5

Narrative Writing and Soulful Metaphors

Commentary on Chapter by Barbara Pizer

Donnel B. Stern

There are several directions I want to go at once in discussing Pizer's chapter. I feel strongly about this paper. It moves me, not just as an analyst but as an everyday reader. This is a lovely piece of writing. The chapter also moves me because it addresses things I happen to be passionate about thinking about. Its subject matter, then, is one thing I want to discuss. But I am also drawn to Pizer's *way* of addressing the things she addresses, her route of access to the things that move me. That is the second topic I shall comment on, and the place where I begin.

The psychoanalytic writing I most appreciate doesn't immediately inspire agreement or disagreement; that comes long after the first reading. Instead, the writing I like best offers an experience. I can lose myself in such writing; I can submerge myself in it. Sometimes this kind of prose is dense and theoretical, in which case the immersion requires powerful and sustained intellectual effort. And sometimes it is more like Pizer's chapter: narrative, allusive, aesthetically rewarding, and literary.

Good writing of the dense variety requires a kind of "plowing through," hard work that requires real commitment and feels deeply satisfying when I'm finished, like a workout at the gym that challenges me right at the limits of what I can do. The risk in that kind of reading is boredom, which is what happens when you give up the commitment to understand but keep reading anyway—that is, you stop making the effort, but you keep going through the motions. That's when you realize that you've read the same sentence or paragraph four times and you still don't know what it says.

The kind of writing Pizer has done here, though, doesn't require me to plow. On the contrary, it requires me to take my hand off the tiller and let the writing wash over me. Rather than penetrating it or pinning it down or getting a fix on it, I need to allow this kind of writing to do whatever *it*

DOI: 10.4324/9781032666303-7

will do to *me*. Actually, the truth is that the same thing happens even with the densest writing, but only after you have been working hard with it for a while. If you really want to make difficult writing your own, if you want to feel that you really understand it, you have to dissolve its difficulty. You have to become so familiar with it that it eventually does to you what more narrative writing does immediately and naturally. Even with dense writing, that is, you have to get to the point where you can allow *it* to have its effect on *you*. But the hard work comes first.

In the case of poetry, or writing like Pizer's in this chapter, the hard work comes later. You have to let the writing have its way with you right off the bat, and then, later on, you can wonder about what you might have taken from it. What has found its way into your mind? This kind of reading requires commitment, too; it's just a different kind of commitment. It's the commitment to freedom of thought, an insistence on allowing whatever will arise by itself in experience. It's a commitment to the unbidden.

In this sense, Pizer's writing is much more like psychoanalysis itself than is dense theoretical writing. In psychoanalysis we try to find our way to new experience. That is the main thing. Only when we have freed ourselves to experience something new can we think about it in a directed, ordered, effortful way. That is what Pizer has told us, in one way or another, throughout this chapter; it was also one of Steve Mitchell's many interests, as Pizer reminds us, and it is one of my own, as well. What matters is the freedom to allow new experience, which requires a commitment to uncertainty and curiosity, a commitment to taking your hand off the tiller, to not knowing where new experience is going to go.

But just as we can lose our way and our commitment with dense material, resulting in boredom, there is a risk attached to reading good narrative psychoanalytic writing, too. If we do not maintain our commitment to the greatest openness and curiosity we can muster, we allow the experience to be too easy, to wash over us with little effect, leaving us with the impression of too little depth. This, too, can be a kind of boredom. That's why poetry and painting sometimes bore us, I think: we don't take the reins off our imagination and give it its head. We need to feel our way through an experience of this kind with a direction and discipline that is nevertheless not the result of the conscious expenditure of effort—something like water finding its way down through a bed of stones. If we don't do that, poetry is nothing more than a pretty-sounding collection of words on the page, and painting is a collection of vaguely interesting marks.

If you want to look at a Rothko painting, you have to stand there and disappear into the painting for a while. In Pizer's chapter, if you were to read or listen without the requisite care, you would end up with the experience of a nice story. The problem we all sometimes have, when we listen to or look at something that is not too difficult to follow, is that we're tempted to shove what we're experiencing into the easiest categories to fulfill, despite the fact that those categories may not be the best fit. Letting yourself get away with the impression that a Rothko looks like a sunset is not going to make you like Rothko. Forcing yourself to focus hard and sharply on the details of a dense stretch of words is very different than remaining open and trying to allow the *words* to reach *you*; yet both are varieties of discipline.

So there are two kinds of good psychoanalytic writing, and the kinds of reading they require are, in a way, mirror images of one another. In the first kind, you have to work hard to read well, and then, later on, you finally arrive at an understanding good enough that you can go back and allow the words and meanings to wash over you. In the second kind, you have to allow your imagination free rein; you have to *begin* by letting the words wash over you; and if you read well and imagine deeply, you may be able to think hard about it later on and understand something differently.

Not everyone seems to agree that both kinds of writing are good for psychoanalysis. Because Freud defined our field as a science, and because ego psychology took that lineage for granted (often with elegance and grace—consider Kris's papers on memory, George Klein on perception, or anything at all by Loewald—but often, too, with scientism and deadly literalness), psychoanalytic writing has far too often been inspired by some kind of allegiance to science. There are those who feel that that traditional scholarly form should be maintained as our sole ideal, just as it stands. More recently, though, some writers have constructed new kinds of theoretical essays, essays that speak to their readers in more affectively immediate terms without sacrificing intellectual rigor. These essays owe more to the style of the *Times Literary Supplement* or *The New Yorker*, or even to certain kinds of continental philosophical writing, than they do to Hartmann or Rapaport. I have tried to work in this vein. And today, it seems, the cutting edge may be in writing that is enthusiastically inspired by literature. Pizer's chapter is part of this latest development.

We need all kinds of writing in psychoanalysis. Why shouldn't we give ourselves the widest kind of license to awaken one another to new experiences of the work we have in common? It is true that we need theory to write in a literary way, because even literary psychoanalytic papers are not exactly literature. They seek to do something different than just tell a story—or, rather, they tell a very particular kind of story, for very particular purposes. Before we can write about psychoanalysis in a literary way, we need to work its ideas so deeply into our minds that we live them. But most of us have done that. Our training, our analyses, and our clinical experience prepare us to write, and read, either way.

I believe our editorial policies should change to allow newer forms of psychoanalytic writing into our journals. There should be a place for both traditional scholarly writing and writing of this narrative, literary kind. In fact, I have had the opportunity to affect editorial policies in just this way. In the journal that I edit (*Contemporary Psychoanalysis*), we have solicited, accepted, and published narrative or literary manuscripts, and we will continue to do so. We would even consider publishing poetry, if we judged that it would awaken in our readers a new experience of doing psychoanalytic work or of thinking about psychoanalysis. We have had a number of poetry submissions, though we have not yet accepted a poem.

I am not alone among psychoanalytic editors in thinking this way. Jody Messler Davies and Neil Altman, coeditors of *Psychoanalytic Dialogues*, have published a panel showcasing new forms of psychoanalytic writing (Panel on Experiments, 2001). But not all editors take this position, I am afraid. I hope that in the future, publishing a wider variety of written psychoanalytic communications will seem valuable to all of us.

Now, on to the content of what Pizer has written. Consider the interests or activities that might serve as examples of Pizer's nonanalytic third. The examples that leap to mind, besides poetry, are things like movies, plays, and novels—new stories to disembed us from the old ones. But we need not limit ourselves to the most obviously narrative arts. I mentioned Mark Rothko. I am something more than I was for having spent several hours at the retrospective of Rothko's work at the Whitney Museum in New York several years ago. Sports, various collecting interests, and any number of other passions serve the same purpose for many of us. But I would hesitate to be too specific about exactly what these passionate interests do for us. And besides, what about those passionate interests of others that don't appeal to me? What about bullfighting, or behavior therapy, or George W. Bush?

The problem here is that any of these pastimes *could* serve as a nonanalytic third; we just wouldn't all agree that they have anything to do with making us better people. Because Pizer has used the work of an estimable poet in her essay, we may think that the nonanalytic third is inevitably some kind of good thing. In fact, its goodness is completely irrelevant. In my way of understanding it, the nonanalytic third is a means by which we create an alternative to an experience in treatment that otherwise just keeps on keeping on. The alternative may be a new perception, or it may just be a different attitude in relating to the old one. Take, for example, Sam's dreams that Pizer rewrote as poetry. Pizer has laid them out as free verse, which has the effect of recontextualizing them in a way that makes you experience them differently than you would have if you had merely heard them read aloud or read them in conventional paragraphs. It gives Sam's dreams a substance I don't think they would have had, at least for me, without this particular visual treatment. The dreams are linked, via the association to poetry, to a different kind of expression and imagination. And so we can say that Pizer's use of her interest or passion in poetry helped her here; but it also helped me. It set what she was discussing, the "figure" of her thinking, against a different ground; and in doing that, what she was discussing became a different figure.

To make the point that a nonanalytic third doesn't have to be something *Good* (with a capital G), let's take an example of a nonanalytic third that isn't necessarily *Bad* but that doesn't have any relevance at all to moral goodness.

Let's take *food*.

I love to eat. I really look forward to every meal and to the various forays in between. I have to stop myself from thinking during the morning about what my favorite takeout place may be preparing for lunch. It is in this vein that you should hear the following vignette, which I also used in my book (D. B. Stern, 1997, pp. 103–111).

I was in the middle of an incredibly sticky enactment with a patient who had been unaccountably furious at me for weeks. I figured out something about what had gone wrong between us, and I communicated it to him. As a result, some of the close bond between us, which had been severely threatened, reappeared. My patient understood that he hadn't seen things very clearly for quite a while. However, he pointed out, it was obvious that I hadn't seen very clearly, either. Why was that, he asked.

I didn't have a very good answer for him. The best I could do, off the cuff, was a gustatory metaphor: I could tell him, I said, that the way I had experienced the situation was as if he had shown me a hardboiled egg in the palm of his hand, representing his implacable rage at me, and had expected me to see that it was not actually a hardboiled egg at all, but an artichoke. That is, I went on, he had showed me rage, expecting me to see that it wasn't rage at all, but hurt feelings. I said that I could tell him nothing more than that it had looked like a hardboiled egg until it suddenly looked like an artichoke. My patient laughed. (That was good, because I really don't know what I would have done if he hadn't.) I don't know that he understood me any better than I understood myself, but at least he was convinced, maybe by the improbability of my metaphor, that I meant what I said. Later on we made more sense of what had happened, but for the time being the meta-phor took up the slack and allowed us to negotiate a difficult moment.

It was a very particular metaphor, wasn't it? Not as profound or mov-ing as Pizer's, but quite particular to me. And it wouldn't have occurred to me without my interest in food. I didn't tell him, after all, that his rage had seemed to be a cat until it was a dog. I didn't say that it looked like water-color until it looked like acrylic (well, that wouldn't have been funny, and I was depending on the humor, after all). I said it seemed like one kind of food until it seemed like another.

Now, of course, I was well aware that the metaphor was ridiculous. As I said, I even counted on the humor to help. But without even thinking about it, I turned to food to make this particular meaning. Food was my nonana-lytic third here.

And so the nonanalytic third can really be any interest or passionate involvement at all, anything that the analyst can use to get a foot in the door, anything that, in suggesting itself to the analyst's mind and opening the way for a new metaphor, makes room for a new perception, a new feel-ing, a new kind of relatedness.

Ah, but here, I think, we get right to the heart of the matter: a new kind of relatedness. It used to be that we thought you changed the transference-countertransference by understanding it. We had the idea that insight usu-ally *preceded* relational change. But in recent decades, that idea seems to have been turned on its head, so that we are now often inclined to believe that *relatedness* must change if *insight* is to occur (e.g., Ghent, 1995; D. N. Stern et al., 1998; D. B. Stern, 2003, 2004). We think of insight less often as the mutative agent and more often as the sign that the important change has already taken place.

Then what *is* the mutative agent? For many of us, it is the negotiation of enactments. We know that the contents of consciousness are heavily influenced by the nature of the interpersonal field. That is, the unformulated meanings to two people of what is happening between them are a prime influence on what they can experience in one another's presence. The unformulated meanings of an enactment limit the explicit meanings that can come about during the enactment. We might even say that this limitation on new meanings is what defines an enactment. An enactment is a rigid state of relatedness in which the experience that would allow an alternative perspective on the interaction is available to neither the analyst nor the patient. To participate unconsciously in an enactment is to unconsciously constrict the curiosity that would make alternative perceptions knowable. And therefore, of course, anything we can do to make an alternative perception more available is good. Alternative perceptions loosen enactment's hold; or rather, alternative perceptions define enactment's demise.

The meanings prevented by enactments are absolutely vital for the analyst and the analysand to find their way into a position to construct. I take the position that the reason we don't formulate experience, when we don't, is that we do not and cannot construct the interpersonal field between us that would allow us to do so. Potential new experience is obscured, that is, by a state of relatedness. Benjamin (1990, 1999, 2000) tells us that the relaxation of enactments, which are doer-done to (sadomasochistic) kinds of integrations, requires the dyad to construct an *analytic* third (the name of this idea, of course, inspired the name of Pizer's), an experience of the relatedness between analyst and patient that is meaningful only in that context and that belongs to neither alone.

So in this sense, Pizer has made a contribution to our thinking about the negotiation of enactments. We find our way to new perceptions of ourselves and our patients by noticing, as we do our work, small affective inconsistencies, gaps and absences in feeling, and other discomforts. It's as if we are walking along a forest path, and our sweaters snag on branches as we pass. We stop and investigate the affective snag, try to untangle it, and in doing so we feel our way deeply enough into the tangle that it sometimes expands into the hint of a previously unsuspected (and unformulated) meaning. Through our openness to affective discomfort—a kind of feelingful chafing—we find ways to allow our curiosity freer play. (For a detailed description of this process, see D. B. Stern, 2003, 2004.)

In this process the nonanalytic third sometimes plays a very important role, because it is from the parts of life we feel most deeply and fondly that we draw our most soulful metaphors. Often, it is by means of these soulful metaphors that the analyst gives voice to affective snags and chafing that, until then, may have been only vaguely meaningful. In other words, sometimes the nonanalytic third, which starts out as an expression completely personal to the analyst, becomes the core around which a new incarnation of the analytic third is built. The personal and nonanalytic morphs into the social and analytic. I think this is what happened when Pizer introduced poetry into the work with Sam.

It is also what happened between my patient and me. The metaphor I used with my patient did not exactly illuminate things, but it did give him a very clear impression that I, too, felt I had to accept that I had been helpless in the grip of my experience. I think my admittedly odd communication helped us find ground from which we could then talk about what our mutual experience had been. Our openness to the nonanalytic third sometimes allows the negotiation of enactments we did not even know were there.

References

Benjamin, J. (1999/1990). Recognition and destruction: An outline of intersubjectivity. In S. A. Mitchell & L. Aron (Eds.), *Relational psychoanalysis: The emergence of a tradition* (pp. 183–200). Hillsdale, NJ: The Analytic Press.

Benjamin, J. (1999). Afterword to "Recognition and destruction: An outline of intersubjectivity." In S. A. Mitchell & L. Aron (Eds.), *Relational psychoanalysis: The emergence of a tradition* (pp. 201–210). Hillsdale, NJ: The Analytic Press.

Benjamin, J. (2000). Intersubjective distinctions: Subjects and persons, recognitions, and breakdowns: Commentary on paper by Gerhardt, Sweetnam, and Borton. *Psychoanalytic Dialogues, 10*, 43–55.

Ghent, E. (1995). Interaction in the psychoanalytic situation. *Psychoanalytic Dialogues, 5*, 479–491.

Dimen, M., Sweetnam, A., & Jones, A.A. (2001). Panel on experiments in new forms of psychoanalytic writing. *Psychoanalytic Dialogues, 11*, 823–890.

Stern, D. B. (1997). *Unformulated experience: From dissociation to imagination in psychoanalysis*. Hillsdale, NJ: The Analytic Press.

Stern, D. B. (2003). The fusion of horizons: Dissociation, enactment, and understanding. *Psychoanalytic Dialogues, 13*, 843–873.

Stern, D. B. (2004). The eye sees itself: Dissociation, enactment, and the achievement of conflict. *Contemporary Psychoanalysis, 40*, 197–238.

Stern, D. N., Sander, L., Nahum, J., Harrison, A., Bruschweiler-Stern, N., & Tronick, E. (1998). Noninterpretive mechanisms in psychoanalytic therapy. *International Journal of Psychoanalysis, 79*, 903–921.

Chapter 6

"Eva, Get the Goldfish Bowl"

Affect and Intuition in the Analytic Relationship[1]

Tacked onto my bulletin board from an old Sunday *New York Times Magazine* is an interview with Jonathan Foer (Solomon, 2005). "Why do I write," it says in bold letters across the top of a double-page spread: "It's not that I want people to think I am smart, or even that I am a good writer. I write because I want to end my loneliness" (p. 43).

Right or wrong, I imagine Foer discovering some crucial or maybe long-forgotten aspects of himself or his experiencing within the characters he conjures, and in these deeply magical moments he becomes accompanied! Similarly, I believe the loneliness that he refers to may be commonplace in our analytic profession, and when we open to the power of our patient's affects, we may be surprised to find a resonant aspect of our self awakening from some dormant place within. I will illustrate such mutual awakening by telling you about my work with Julian and an accidental happenstance that led me to develop what I call an *outrageous interpretation*.

Julian

The man I call Julian was referred to me some years ago. Although it was made clear that he was a scientist of world renown, I had no idea why he was coming or what I would find when I opened the door of my office and saw him sitting there in the waiting room. A professor in his mid-fifties, he wore a denim work shirt and blue jeans held up by wide, bright-red suspenders that almost matched his bushy red hair. Could this be the guy I was meant to see? He looked up with a shy smile and melancholy eyes. I saw in this figure a mixture of Gregory Peck and Huckleberry Finn.

"Julian?" I queried.

He nodded.

"Please come in."

DOI: 10.4324/9781032666303-8

Julian is the second of four boys, born of an affectionate woman, Julia, who despite her superior intellect and high ambition postponed a career until the last of her children was grown, not only for the sake of mothering them and providing the stability of a home, but also in order to nurture a well-known, driven husband whose demanding profession took much time, travel, family moves, and energy. Dr. G is an energetic man himself, both generous and stingy to a fault, adoring of his kids and taking them on great adventures while simultaneously tending to his own needs first and assuming an earned right of residence at the center of his world. But Dr. G was never a snob, merely a loving and impossible man with a hair-trigger temper. And, indeed, brilliant. I imagine that all of his kids carry a similar potential for success. However, Conrad, the eldest, suffered a severe break in his late-teen years, and Michael, eighteen months younger than Julian, was killed in a car accident during his sophomore year at college. Ben, the youngest, perhaps the sweetest of the boys, fell out of his crib and onto his head at a very early age. Although doctors have claimed it doubtful that this fall is at all connected to his severe learning disabilities, Julia has always held herself responsible.

For good or ill, Julia tends to take responsibility for the fate or shortcomings or perceived needs of others, particularly her loved ones, which may be related to the fact that Ben—due to his mother's steadfast devotion to tutoring and special care—has surpassed all expectation in the learning department. However, given all the turmoil, pain, and hardship as well as love and fun and adventure in this family, Julian was and remains the realized prodigy among his brothers. And given his stunning successes and quick temper, he readily accepts the attribution that he is "just like his father."

The first time I understood this was when Julian set out for us his initial set of instructions for our enterprise: "I'm too arrogant and I've come to fix my marriage."

Julian made it clear to me that this chore was entirely up to him. He loved his four girls deeply, and he loved how his wife, Carrie, took such wonderful care of them. He loved to watch her eyes when she was with them. "But I'm out of the loop," he says. "She never looks at me that way."

"How come?" I ask.

"Because I'm arrogant. I get mad. I work too much."

"Is that what the kids say?" I want to know.

"The kids love me. We have a wonderful time together. But they parrot what their mother says. Especially the second oldest."

"What do you think?" I asked Julian.

As if to erase the question, he briefly turns his head to the side, sliding out of contact, and then he said, "Well, about my work, there's one more thing . . . (pause). Sometimes when I'm talking about it to a colleague, or even in a public lecture, I find myself getting teary. The crying, it just comes over me without notice."

As Julian pauses to gather in his thoughts, I see the rims of his eyes go red and tears forming at their outer corners. "And?" I query.

"Or when my kids say something meaningful, or if I'm repeating what happened with them to Rich—he's a really good friend, I can start to tear up with no warning at all. I can't seem to control it. I need to learn how not to do that."

"Learn not to cry?" I asked.

"Yes. It's too embarrassing."

"Well, if that is really one of your major goals, I'm sorry, Julian," I replied. "Because whatever work may be possible between us, I can promise you right now I'll never be able to help you with that one."

He sat there silent. So did I.

Before I tell you why and why not my comment to Julian is what I have come to call an *outrageous interpretation*, I need to say something about affect and the analyst's subjectivity and tell you some things about me and the goldfish bowl.

Affect and the Analyst's Subjectivity

Today, people who know me well understand my tendency to become intimidated by certain types of "brilliant mind." Feeling intimidated is distinct from, but often leads to, the other more highly charged state in which I suddenly and literally "go dumb."

The roots of what I am trying to tell you go way back. I come from a fairly close-knit family with four girls. Not surprisingly, each of us played out our designated roles in the family system. My older sister, Ilse, an avid reader, math and science whiz, skipped several grades at school, and whenever, in my half-blind, dyslexic way, I reached a classroom where she had skated through, the teacher greeted me with songs of her praise and predictions for me of which I would invariably fall short. My sister—with eyelids at half-mast and glancing sideways—faithfully tried to tutor me in those subjects, predicting all the while that should I pass my chemistry regents exam, *it would be a miscarriage of justice*. At school and at home, Ilse was cool and easy compared to my tantrums. Unflappable. She shunned confrontation of any kind yet somehow managed to get what she wanted even if she had to sneak it, like the comic books underneath her bed. Somehow I was convinced that Ilse held the key to mother's heart, and no matter how hard I tried to be like her, I could never manage it. Thus I became the queen of "back-talk," fought with my younger sister (despite the seven-year gap between us), stood up for the baby, and focused on more outrageous underground activities—like filching coins from mother's purse with which to buy her little presents. Although I brought my parents to the edge of despair on more than one occasion, I also held the reputation of a generous, expressive, and warm-hearted soul who could not bear the suffering of others or give up on what I considered to be a just cause. I would burst into tears at the drop of a hat.

Family dinner-table conversations were high-spirited affairs. Often my Dad would introduce a subject, offer an opinion, and invite us to debate. The younger set appeared content to mainly listen until a place was made for them to take their turn. The same rule, however, did not apply to Ilse and me. Not being as quick-witted as she is, I often felt unable to articulate my thoughts in the time I perceived was allotted. But it was more than that. At the time, I had no idea that I was being raised in a Cartesian culture in which "intellectual pursuits" were highly valued and "emotional reactions" carried no cachet. Yet for me it felt impossible to conceive of acceptably "logical" or "rational" explanations for what, in my heart, I just "knew" to be true, and in these situations, I ceased to speak, and my lower lip would begin to wobble. Whenever this happened, father would immediately look across the table to his wife with a mocking sigh. "Eva, get the goldfish bowl, Barbara is going to cry again."

I can still retain a sense of that inexplicable "spacing out" that seems to occur between the silence of intimidation and the actual releasing of tears. There are no words. And all I can say about it is that it feels like a drop. A little terror in the stomach—like when a rising elevator all of a sudden *stops*.

"Eva, get the goldfish bowl, Barbara is going to cry again!" Today it's clear to me that his comment was meant to lighten up his own tension at the table.

Today I can more readily bind up those regions of wordlessness where I feel stunned into silence by someone's quick-witted intellectualizing.

Mostly, I can allow myself a moment's mental pause to gather my bearings when I'm intimidated instead of racing headlong toward that drop into the rabbit hole where I disappear entirely. I can recognize that feeling intimidated is a state in me that signals a shift, sending me plummeting into the dark land of dumb beyond existence. So now that hindsight helps me at least to distinguish these two separate self-states, I feel more able to recognize the difference between a brilliant mind and an intellectual gymnast. Going dumb for me is deeper in the body, deeper in childhood, boundless, a sucking down, a consequence of undercurrent—the outcome of whatever seemed to me so present in that dining room but never spoken.

Ironically, going dumb was more accurately a cover-up for outrage over being misperceived or teased for a mode of procedural experiencing that was alien in my family, out of bounds, forbidden. There was something forbidden about being "too much"—too much picking up on the unspoken, too much sensitivity, too much emotion, too much caring about another person's feelings. "Eva, get the goldfish bowl!"

I think, at this point, it would not be out of line to conjecture that my spacing out the title of Jonathan Foer's interview from *The New York Times* may be related in some way to the business of going dumb. The title, if you would like to know, is "The Rescue Artist."

Outrageous Interpretations

My rapidly uttered, unequivocal guarantee not to help Julian control the flow of his tears might be considered the first of a number of outrageous interventions I have made in our first five years together. Outrageous because at this juncture I had hardly met the man. My inquiry was minimal. I had full awareness of what I was saying and yet no conscious idea of what the words meant to me, to whom I was talking, or what impact such a statement might have on us. Outrageous because in my analytic work, it is unusual for me to foreclose that quickly with such minimal analytic tact.

So perhaps we were both surprised. I do not know. *But here is the belief that is central to my thesis.* My comment was born, or perhaps articulated, through a mutual unconscious process that took place between Julian and me, a process that began first in my own history and then emerged in interaction with Julian and constituted for me a bridge across the gap between intimidation and going dumb. I believe that bridge in turn provided a bridge between the analyst and the scientist, an accident of fate that grew into my forming a theoretical/technical concept that I call the *outrageous interpretation.*

Even though it was more than forty years ago, I vividly recall my clinical internship in which the delivery of "a good interpretation" was a triumph devoutly to be wished. In that collegial culture of Grand Rounds, the interpretation was regarded as a valued object, the "thing" that promoted "therapeutic action," a product of our superior thinking that we "gave" to our patients for their edification and growth.

Now I want to be clear that even today I see nothing wrong with genuine offerings from time to time. Call them interpretations if you like. I'm not immune to interpretive behavior when I believe it might be just the tool we need to move the treatment forward. Similarly, I may consider something that I say to the person sitting in the patient's place will serve as a Bionian container or a Winnicottian opening of potential space in moments of trauma or doubt; and I am very at home with Lewis Aron's (1992) notion of interpretation as an expression of the analyst's subjectivity as a way of adjusting the relationship.

But in addition to these, Julian has brought out in me yet another mode of intervention that is not merely an "inadvertent disclosure" (Aron, 1992; B. Pizer, 1997), not just what could be seen as an "enactment" (Bromberg, 1998; Davies, 1999; McLaughlin, 1991; D. B. Stern, 1997), or a simple answer to Mitchell's (2000) provocative declaration that it is important, in certain instances, to take a subjective position. Nor is what I'm talking about exactly like Ogden's (1994) "interpretative action" in which the verbal content occurs *inside* of the analyst. All of the above does have a place or space in the overall schema of the work I do. But here I refer to a specifically contextual declarative statement that appears to eschew my usual sense of analytic decorum while simultaneously seeming to reflect some out-of-the-ordinary or mutually forbidden aspect in the intersubjective moment. I suddenly get an uncanny sense of "knowing" that my analytic partner and I do both really "know" what we don't allow ourselves to know we know. Furthermore, the mysterious contents are almost less important than the process of disallowing knowledge, of not knowing how we come to not know we know it.

What I found with Julian, or became aware of, triggered by the intersubjective interactions between us, was a mode of intervention born of the analyst's apperception of a dissociated space within her patient that suddenly resonates with a heretofore dissociated space within herself—generating a spontaneous verbal gesture that delivers fresh affective energy into the field between them.

I propose that an *outrageous interpretation* is a rapid two-step process describing creative use of previously dissociated experiencing, a process that may be common to many analysts.

While in my case the term *outrageous* refers to a personal response of rebellious outrage triggered by something in the present situation that brings back early dissociated shame for once having opened up my heart or my mouth, it becomes an outrageous interpretation when that response with its accompanying affects is *transformed* into a contextually relevant intervention, a direct translation aimed at delivering affective energy into the clinical moment, with the express purpose of disrupting or dismantling ossified dissociative patterns in both myself and my patient.

In other words, the interpretive aspect of my outrageous intervention reflects a freshly created transformation of intense shame over affective responsiveness that my going dumb repeatedly shuts down. Ironically, there may be nothing particularly outrageous in the newly shaped content of what I end up saying to my patient. It's the tone, the pressured inflection so out of keeping with the words that I uncharacteristically allow to come out, emerging from a dissociated place in me and bearing enough affective intensity to enter a place in my patient (Julian) that has also been shut down, so that he too may regain a state of presence and affective experience. Now invoking Freud's (1912) recognition of the unconscious in one person communicating directly to the unconscious in the other, I arrive at a general speculation, as already suggested, that an outrageous interpretation may be a message transmitted from an affectively dissociated place in the analyst to an affectively dissociated place in the patient.[2]

If the message were simply a dissociated enactment, it would be simply outrageous. To be an outrageous interpretation, the charged message must be transformed to suit the patient's emergent affective experience and availability for analytic contact and process.

If we wish to categorize the outrageous interpretation as an "analytic technique," I would say that the "technique" occurs before the analyst's utterance. The "technique" involves the analyst's openness to knowing one's patient in the context of ongoing and emergent self-discovery, having developed a good alliance and a tentative working formulation of why or how affects are "stuck" in the patient and also in the analyst. For example, with a trauma survivor stuck in an acute phase of relating to the analyst

through repeated sadomasochistic behaviors, the analyst's outrageous interpretation may be the outcome of some affective arrow (from the patient's
dissociations) that has broken through the analyst's skin and reached a
trauma trigger in the analyst's "forgotten" past. So the intervention usually
carries with it a definite setting of limits delivered in the imperative mode,
a containing "reality check" that functions paradoxically to tie up loose
ends in both analyst and patient. Thus, affects held in dissociation have the
potential to be acknowledged, shared in words, and thus move forward.

By strictest definition then, my first outrageous interpretation with Julian
may more aptly be considered an enactment or an inadvertent disclosure
(see Chapter 2). I had a strong intuitive sense of who he was but no supporting data yet. However, I did know for sure that I could never succeed
in teaching him not to cry. Mine was a gut response. I had not yet built
a theoretical, technical construct that might provide a definition for what
many of us know we do with certain patients at certain times. Naming the
behavior as an outrageous interpretation may serve to guide our spontaneity
in a more disciplined way, setting it apart from the norm, giving us a speakable term for evaluating the usefulness of such a move.

Finally, I want to emphasize specifically that an outrageous interpretation
is actually the outcome of a highly disciplined mode of mindful, creative
engagement primarily geared to *grab onto, hold, and move affect forward*.[3]
In Julian's case, I now see clearly why I delayed telling you the area of his
expertise. His field involves a study of the universe, in particular, the nature
of black holes.

My View from the Bridge: Between Julian and Me

1.   Grabbing On

As I engage in the analytic enterprise, I try hard to disabuse myself of the
tempting notion that I can ever fully or fairly fathom the nature of activity
within a marriage as reported to me by my patient. However, I can say that I
found Julian's set picture of his interactions with Carrie—blow-ups and punishments, "unprecedented" rages, and cold retreats—rather startling on two
counts: the first being that Carrie and Julian both accepted the attribution that
he was the bad guy, which related to the second idea that he alone could fix it.

There was something both "smooth" and intractable about Julian's presentation, or maybe also something mesmerizing in my own sense of his

melancholy over the lonely burden that he took into himself. These two intractable assumptions that Julian carried—ultimate responsibility for the breakdown in his marriage and the need to change himself for his wife and the family—occupied the major portion of our focus over the first year and a half. Looking back, I can identify four interventions that helped me to challenge his stuck sense of certainty. Although the interpretations I refer to might well have contained a grain of truth, even at the time of delivery they struck me as so indefensibly *outrageous* that I felt myself float over the black hole of intimidated dumbness. I should say that prior to the first of these four happenings, we had begun to build a bridge of trust in one another, some sense of play. After all, he accepted my initial refusal to help him stop his tears; he did come back.

Over time, Julian opened up to dreaming, became aware of how his incessant worrying might somehow be connected to vulnerability and loss. His rendering of memories around growing up, his acknowledging the unaccountable relentlessness of rules that governed his adult behavior, and his willingness to wonder about all of this with me invited my participation.

First dream: Julian dreamed he was in the new home of a former roommate from college who shares Julian's particular field in science and who seems to be enjoying his second marriage. Inside and out, his new place is warm and beautiful. Real or imagined, Julian describes how the house in his dream is built. "There is a rock overhang that serves as its roof and is attached by a beam. The house could shift. I worry about what would happen to the windows. But my roommate says that it's okay, we can accommodate the fix."

I ask for associations. Julian has none.

"The rock," I say, "the overhang. It's rigid and the house is flexible. I wonder what part of you might be rigid and what part flexible?"

"Taking care of Carrie after her surgery," he replies. "Doing the drains and dressings. I know I followed the post-op instructions to a tee. But she would always stop me and say I was hurting her; she'd say I was doing it all wrong. I could never do anything enough or good enough for her." Julian sighs. "But the way she treated me—it became an obligation. I want you to know," he emphasized, "I really love to tend to people. Ask any of my students. But Carrie, she kept telling me I was wrong. I ended up yelling at her, 'I'm doing it right, Carrie, look the other way!' And then Sara would hear me yelling and say, 'Don't be mean to Mommy,' and she'd call to the other three, 'Daddy made Mommy cry.'"

Julian tells me that he's a stoic when he's sick. "Carrie says I'm unsympathetic when it comes to illness. She accuses me of not caring and thinking only of myself. She says I don't contribute to the household, that I go off on these trips and leave her doing all the work. Even when I'm home, she says, she's the one who has to get up and drive the kids to school. Well, I don't think she has to get up."

Now I hear Julian arguing with himself. "Just because they ask her for a ride. I don't think it's good for them. I think they're old enough to walk."

I am quiet.

"Is it rigid to have rules for kids?" he continues. "Carrie says I make too many rules. Don't you think a ten-year-old is adult enough to walk or take the bus for no more than a mile from home?"

I notice that my mind is going blank.

"What do you think?" Julian repeats his question—more emphatically this time. "Carrie thinks I'm just like my dad—self-involved—and maybe I am."

"*Or maybe not,*" I retort outrageously, mentally shaking myself free. "*Maybe you're involved in handing over to Carrie feeling bad about yourself so you don't have to deal with your own guilt. So you don't need to do anything, and she can do the work of punishing you with her words.*"

Tears begin to form in the corners of Julian's eyes.[4] And by now I take his tears as overflow from having touched some feeling by surprise, a feeling that in turn most surely touches me.

A few months later, Julian asks me why it is that he stays up at night worrying about things that don't make sense to worry about. When I ask him to elaborate, he says he worries about his favorite mentee who is about to accept an offer from another prestigious university, and Julian doesn't want to let him go. He will miss him. He believes it would be better for the guy's career to stay where he is, but at the same time it would be wrong to try too hard to convince him of it.

"I remember," Julian recalls, "the colleagues who wined and dined me and convinced me I'd do well to come here. And I have. I've made *xx* theory my area of expertise. I'm well known for it."

"And then," as if untouched by his fame, he goes on to say, "I stay up all night worrying that all the post-docs who interviewed here won't come—will choose somewhere else."

I ask whether Julian could elaborate further about his feelings of being known.

The question causes him to redden around the eyes. "Nobody ever asked me that." There is a pause. "It's an issue for Carrie, my being well known in the world," Julian brushes at his face with a hand. "Carrie doesn't feel known by me, so she won't acknowledge me when I come home. No kiss hello or goodbye or goodnight."

"You mean tit for tat."

"Yes. But it isn't true that I don't want to listen to her. I try. But she stops me when I don't get it right away. And when I try to tell her something about my day, she rolls her eyes in disgust, or she corrects my grammar."

We sit silently together.

"In front of the kids," he continues. "She undermines me with the kids."

When it seems he has no more to say, I begin to think out loud. "Seems to me, Julian, you know two kinds of recognition. Your oldest girls and your little one, they get 100% on a test, they look at their score, and they're not surprised. They already know they're good. And then there's Sara. You say she gets attention because she 'waves her arms around' until she's seen. How is it for you?"

Julian doesn't hesitate. "In the world I get both kinds but I choose the first. I spent fifteen years waving my arms around about my ideas. Fifteen years knowing I was right while people didn't believe me, put me down, put up with me. But I kept waving my arms around. Now that I have both kinds of recognition, I've promised myself never to complain again!"

"You mean, feel a need for something?" I query.

"People just don't ask me that." Julian weeps. "I miss my good friend Rich. He's an eccentric and he's ten years older than me. A musician. Everybody loves him. Rich has always been there for me, and I've tried to be there for him. His Mom is dying now, so he's gone out to live with her. I need him but he won't let himself need me. We used to have lunch together three times a week. He used to come and give my kids piano lessons."

I know that Julian doesn't like what's showing on his face. He turns away. In myself I'm looking for my own goldfish bowl. The last thing I want to do is embarrass this man. And so to balance out the flood of sorrow in my tone, I say outrageously, *"Could be you need Carrie and rules to keep the mess of all those feelings that you have in line."*

In the next session, as if no time had passed, Julian begins to speak as he walks in the door.

"My mother needed me and I couldn't give her what she needs" (sic). He settles in and continues. "My older brother, Conrad, lost it after high school,

and Michael, only eighteen months younger than me, died at twenty-four.
I remember when we were living in New Haven. I was ten and completely
occupied with wondering about what is 'the meaning of life?' When I was
twelve, I recognized that I could break the rules and my parents couldn't
stop me. They had no control. I palled around with all the hoodlums, I stole
money from my mother, I stole from stores. I spent two days in jail. And
all that while I was getting along with the smart good guys, getting along
with the teachers. Skipped seventh grade. I did well at school. At twelve
and thirteen, it was sex and drugs. I skipped twelfth grade and the final year
of high school. I graduated with Conrad. At fourteen I found Buddhism.
We were living up here then. Spent a month in the summer by myself on
a mountaintop in Maine with nothing but a garbage bag in case it rained.
I had a drawing pad, a pencil, and allowed myself two matches a day. No
sex. That was quite a rule! I had a knife, can opener, some food, a few other
things—not much else."

"How did you get to the mountain?" I asked.

"By that time we had a summer place that all of us love. My parents and
the rest of the family were up there and they dropped me off. Picked me up
when the month was up."

"Were you scared?"

"No."

"Lonely? Did you feel lonely?"

"Yes and no."

"But your parents—they let you do that. On a mountain by yourself?"

"They knew they couldn't stop me. When we were in New Haven," Julian
continued, "my mother hit me and I hit her back. When my father came
home, he took me to his study and said, 'You never hit your mother!' He
pulled off his belt and started to whip me. I picked up his favorite Steuben
vase and said, 'if you come near me, I'll break it.' I jumped out the study
window and was gone for two days."

"Must have been lonely then," I remark.

Once again teary, Julian moves on to tell me how he resonated with
what we talked about last time, how he looks for worries to ground him. He
spoke to his eldest daughter too harshly last night, for forgetting the house
rules, and she sobbed.

"That was probably not too good," I sympathize. "But on the other hand
. . . I wonder what it feels like to her when she's all over the place and soon
to leave for college on her own. I wonder if she feels grounded at all."

"I know that she loves me," Julian says. "We do a lot together. She likes to talk with me about her courses."

A day after this conversation, we are in early summer now, Julian brings us fragments from two dreams:

> *"A valuable granite stone in the shape of a boat—an archeological thing in the ground. Carrie breaks it up. I get mad. She says, 'that's the only way I could get it out of the ground!'"*
>
> *"The other fragment is a fireplace. There's a hanging rack with antique pots... a brass kettle, much like my missing brass flowerpot."*

Julian shifts. I don't know what is dream and what is association. "Carrie says she threw it away. I get mad. Sara comes in with it, holding it. 'It's okay, Dad,' she says."

Then Julian associates to Michael's gravestone at his parents' summer house. He and Carrie got married at the summer house. The brass pot is like his mother's at the summer house. Yesterday he had a fight with Carrie, who made Father's Day plans without consulting him so now they have to renege on their annual invitation to spend the day at his roommate's beach place in Rhode Island. When he confronts Carrie, he says she gets defensive—"hurls the book" at him about how awful he is. It's okay, he thinks to himself. He'll go with Sara.

I don't respond. Julian knows I get uncomfortable when his anger goes underground...

He associates to his old office. A maintenance man came in to repair something and ended up splattering paint all over the walls. "I try to get the head of maintenance to fix it but I can't get him. My secretary comes in. She says she'll take care of it."

"Do you think she can, Julian?" My query is rhetorical. We both seem to be preparing ourselves for what I am about to say. *"Your sense of Carrie's neglect and punishment is the closest you can get to handling the accidental mess you made. It's a mess all right. I think maybe Carrie acts mean to you because somewhere she has to know that you don't love her. What else is there for her to do?"*

The following session, Julian continues wondering with me about his dream. "The rowboat," he ponders, "people sit next to each other in a rowboat... There was an image in the dream where my mother is helping Carrie break it up... "

"Yes?" I encourage him to wonder on.

"About Michael in the dream. It's his gravestone. When Michael died, I wanted to provide for my family, to make up for Michael. Michael liked Carrie better than the other girlfriends I had. I wanted to make up for . . . Carrie wasn't ready to have children. It was me who pressured her. I don't think she ever forgave me for that. It was wrong. I had to have four children to make up for Michael . . ."

And so I conclude what I had begun to say outrageously the day before— neither with the intent to maintain a truth I could not as an outsider claim to know, nor with the hope that I could ever contain what was splattered across the walls of Julian's heart. It wasn't up to me to mess around with the potential breakup of a marriage that I couldn't fairly fathom. My efforts were focused on an attempt to connect a heretofore dissociated space with affective energy. I needed to cry.

"A rowboat and a gravestone, stuck in the ground," I mused. *"Tell me, Julian, how do you take it up and hold it together at the same time? Could it be true that you don't love her, and that's what makes you keep on feeling so bad?"*

2. Holding

In this phase of work, we may experience several fine distinctions. There is a difference between holding and holding on in the grabbing sense. Also, I have come to see how "absolute certainty" acts as camouflage in areas of ambiguous self-esteem and therefore blocks off affect.

Despite Julian's frequent reports of high-volume rages, I don't believe that rages, loudly and explicitly delivered, worry me half as much as they worry him. It's the anger that goes underground that frightens me, the seething kind that you can't see coming. And so far Julian's outbursts have not declared themselves in quite that fashion in my consulting room. But his "absolute certainty" might be a variant.

Most often when absolute certainty registers across the pattern of my mind map, I receive the fallout somewhere to the right of going dumb. It strikes me as less harmful, because it's met with less awareness on my part and dealt with quickly by compliance. Not so, I find, in interactions of this kind with Julian. He kind of hunkers down and sticks it to me in a way I can't escape.

Julian is telling me of a new kind of dream he had after a fun-filled party in his department. He dreams he's at the summer house, on a warm night with a full moon, lying right there in the grass with his academic fellows! (I note that his fellows are both male and female—some of them quite attractive.) They are all together, close, and next to each other and they go to sleep.

Julian has assured me more than once that he would never sleep with a fellow or anyone else outside of his relationship with Carrie. It's not a matter of morality or even happiness, but rather the rules of marriage. And because that behavior is against the rules of marriage, he has never allowed himself the pleasure or freedom of having fantasies. And what about intimacy, I wonder. Are there rules for intimacy?

Julian continues with his dream. "So I'm lying there in the grass with my fellows and I wake up. I see the big barn. A white horse peeks out of the top window of the barn. Then he goes back in again. And then I see him and he *jumps!* He lies there stunned and terribly bloody . . . and finally gets up and goes on."

And now I associate to Julian's adolescent years, his jumping out the window and running away, and his telling me that his parents couldn't stop him. I wonder how he ever found his way back home.

When I ask Julian for his associations, he says, "My mother's favorite grey horse, Laddie. He got gored right in front of the house by a cow. That's when she finally got rid of the cattle that I asked her not to sell because without the cattle I would have to go out and cut the weeds—*me* having to cut those weeds. It would be my job to do. Mother was very upset. She loved Laddie. It was all my fault. I'm guilty for not wanting to cut the weeds."

And now we have arrived at the place where I must illustrate the fine distinction between an outrageous interpretation and an enactment, namely a particular enactment over which I still feel shame. Over the last few weeks, Julian had retreated into an old way of being—covering himself with a blanket of guilt so that I could not get near him. (Only later would I be able to own that I felt impatient and left out.) The hour had come to an end, and I experienced myself as oddly blocked and helpless. It seemed like I could not get through to either one of us and could not sit with the guilt and the shame that I felt Julian experiencing. Against my better judgment, I lend him a paper I have written about holding on and letting go, about intimate relating and the freedom to feel one's feelings while still taking responsibility. I couldn't wait for him to get there on his own.

The next day Julian comes in to tell me (outrageously) that he read the paper as my relating to him my confusion. He is certain that now I have crossed a line! He is panicked. But not too panicked to talk about it.

"My mother," he tells me, "was always needing *me* when what I wanted was to be taken care of."

Suddenly, sitting with Julian, I am seven years old, transported to my Grandma Oppenheimer's farm. . .

"Do you think," I say to Julian, "I am looking for you to take care of me?"

"Absolutely." Julian is locking on. "That is clear."

. . . in the summer that my younger sister was about to be born, Ilse and I are sent away. We spend the entire month of July at Grandma's farm, which would be lots of fun if both my parents were along. . .

"I wanted unconditional love from you," Julian is telling me, "But not from *you*. From a nonperson. Being a person crossed the line."

A hideous Nanny is hired to accompany us. We hate her. She spends her time reading or on the phone.

"Being a person crosses the line."

. . .It is shockingly hot that summer at Grandma's farm. I can feel the heat in my cheeks. There's a stream in the front meadow where we are not supposed to go. We are not allowed to cross the road. We can see the stream from the window of the farmhouse. Ilse and I, we wriggle through the forbidden barbed-wire fence of that front meadow, and we are walking through the high grass. . .

Julian asks me what this issue of intimacy between us that I write about is supposed to mean. What do I want from him? What am I *really* saying?

Silence is useless; Julian will not yield.

Ilse is balancing on a log across the stream when it happens. . .

"My mother paid more attention to my brothers and her best friend's kids. They were always at the house. When I ask her about it, she tells me that I seemed so happy as a child, so self-sufficient. Didn't need anything."

I must have stepped squarely in a nest of yellow jackets.

"I know my mother needs me. It looks like you do too but why won't you admit it? Why else would you give me that paper?"

Julian doesn't raise his voice. But he is fixed on me. He says he is certain that he knows what he is talking about. Why would I not admit what I need from him?

A nest of yellow jackets. A million of them. They swarm around me without mercy. Ilse is screaming bloody murder, but even I can hardly hear her over the sound of the bees.

"She needs me. You do too."

I stand there frozen as the bees narrow in on me and settle on my skin. The more I try to brush them off, the harder they hunker down. I wonder if they know I'm shaking.

I make no argument with Julian. Yet as I sit there, gradually my awareness shifts.

I have no idea how we managed to shimmy back under the barbed-wire fence, fly over the forbidden road, and somehow make it back to the house. But I can feel the terror in my stomach—not only from the bees but from anticipating the sound and sorry scolding that we would most certainly receive for having broken the rules. Broken the rules.

I have no words, nor do I want them in this moment.

Now I am lying on my Grandma's bed, and I can literally feel the cool of a liquid white unguent that she dabs both gingerly and firmly on each red mound of skin. She is humming, humming, humming.

I am amazed by the forgiveness. There never was a scolding, and I got a shiny silver dime for each and every sting.

Now I am able to breathe again.

Two sessions later, Julian presents me with two sheets of lined notebook paper on which he has written a dream from the night before. I am particularly struck by its concluding fragment:

I am with a woman crouching (praying?) beside a large bed, trying to accomplish something. Far away a wizard sends a spell at us. It arrives in the form of a sparkling dust cloud swirling overhead. The specks of dust turn into bees, touch me, and turn me into a bee. I whisper to the woman, "I still love you even though I've been turned into a bee." The End.

I do not immediately ask for associations. Over the next months, Julian relates to me all the ways in which he never felt supported and, it falls out of his mouth, "I don't let anyone support me. Clearly, it's too dangerous."

"The trouble with your certainty," I say to Julian, "is that it may be safe, but it narrows your vision."

Julian shows no evidence of taking that in. But it just occurs to me that it's the same thing with uncertainty, the wobbly kind that hangs out around intimidation, and lingers on the way to going dumb.

"I had this dream I really believed in," he continues, "but by the end I felt it was just wrong."

I don't know if this is an actual dream or a waking nightmare, but he goes on to tell me how he spent his whole young lifetime looking for the answers and they always turned out wrong. "My father was too busy working and my mother spent all her time helping others. I know she loves me, but she doesn't think that I might need her." I tell Julian, as it has just occurred to me, that of all the children, his name sounds like a variant of his mother's name, Julia. I wonder what he makes of that. My mind has thawed. I'm thinking of his earlier dream and that my name begins with B, but I keep that to myself for now.

Another dream: *Julian is lying on his bed. I come to cradle his head to see if he is crying. He turns around to face me. I turn into Carrie; Carrie turns into his mom.*

Then there is a long series of dreams about crime and punishment and the fixed assumption that he is his brother Michael's murderer. We note the many ways that he carries responsibility "just like his mother." His mother, it turns out, cries a lot.

Over time, the fixed assumption that Julian is only like his father softens through continuing recognition of his maternal identifications, and as he allows his fantasies to flourish, so does his reflective functioning.

But growth is never simple or linear, of course. The best we can ever hope for is that affect continues to move forward.

"Maybe if I can make Carrie be less mean to me, I wouldn't want to leave her," Julian hypothesizes.

"Well," I retort outrageously, "maybe you can make her be *more* mean, then you wouldn't have to feel so guilty about how bad you are for even thinking such a thing."

3.   Moving Affect Forward

Julian tells me, "It's like walking a tightrope. If you don't believe what you are doing is right, you will never persevere to the end. On the other hand, if you are too fixed in your views, you will get stuck at a dead end. There is no sure-fire formula. This is the hardest thing to teach my students."

Now this revelation belongs entirely to him. I am smiling to myself.

So we have come a long way, Julian and I. And even though we are not done, here is where we've gotten. In closing, and before I ask some questions of my own, I will relate to you the essence of our final two sessions before a long break, before Julian leaves on his sabbatical abroad.

"So I'm having dinner with Rich, to say good-bye." Julian pauses to give me a little background about what he's going to tell me. "Rich and I, we've had a thing since I was in college. I describe to him the different colors of my sadness. I have a black sadness that's always been a part of me."

Getting back to the present narrative, Julian continues. "I'm telling Rich over coffee that I'm feeling my black sadness. I ask him if I break up with Carrie and move out, does he think it will go away? And he bursts into hysterical laughter. 'I think you'll continue to enjoy life!' he says."

"Do you think so, Julian?"

"Yes. The black sadness is a part of me that isn't gonna go away no matter what I do," he replies. "But I do enjoy life in many different ways."

"Are you thinking of anything in particular?"

"I think both my parents wanted me to complete something they couldn't complete themselves." Julian's voice trails off into further thought. "My parents had handicaps of various kinds. My mother, she's the saintly type."

He trails off again.

"And?" I urge.

"I remember when I was fifteen, looking for the Buddha and spiritual enlightenment. Then I decided I wasn't going to get it. Just now I had the thought that my children would figure it out and explain it to me."

At this moment, mulling over Julian's black sadness, it suddenly occurs to me, *"That's your work isn't it, Julian, to show that you can get out of the black hole?"*

"No," he says, *"to find out if you can get out of the black hole.* I think maybe I'll be able to do that."

"Black holes, from what I understand," I go on, "destroy all information. Whereas black sadness carries useful information. It would be a shame to get rid of it."

Julian's voice leans forward. "You mean, you could *use* the information?"

"Yes." I am surprised by the affirmation in my tone.

But there is a PS. Julian, undaunted by the end of an hour, comes in the next day to set me straight about one important thing.

"It's not about what gets *out* of a black hole," he informs me. "It's what is *in* a black hole. There's a well-known scientist named Hawking, who said there's nothing there. Some people believed it—some didn't at all. Whether they believed it or not *depended on how they looked at it.*"

"But," Julian asserts, "the thing is *they thought they knew. They thought they knew they were right.*"

"And you?"

"I thought that I didn't think that," Julian replies, "I thought that I didn't know. But I wanted to know."

Julian tells me that if you look at it in a different way, not only is there not nothing in a black hole, but as much as you can fit in a small space!

He leaves us with much to ponder. The nothing is something, and not just something, but a lot of it.

The Rescue Artist

So here are the questions that give me pause and that I want to leave with you. Can we ever fully know the places where we live before we have the words? And how is it that for many of us in the helping professions, we can find solace and understanding for others and yet we seem to have so little idea of how to ask for what we need for ourselves? There is a tendency to work so hard at helping that we're in danger of arriving at a way of being in the world that looks to others like we don't need a thing. And that's how we are liable to get sucked in by how we appear to others—leaving us to fall into the well of our own loneliness and/or frenetic activity.

But my work with Julian brought home to me another option. What I mean to say is this: Beyond our own analysis, our patients may awaken in us long-dormant memories of shame and pain and joy, experiences that serve—for a brief time—to cut through loneliness, experiences that may well vitalize, enrich, and enliven who we are and who we've come to be.

So, metaphorically speaking, if Julian is right, and "nothing" is actually a great abundance of "something," and if we were given the choice of two possible structures in which we could contain these mysterious contents — that black hole or the goldfish bowl, I hope I would still opt for the gold-fish bowl. What about you?

Notes

1 An earlier version of this chapter was first presented in 2005 at the Toronto Institute for Contemporary Psychoanalysis, Toronto, Canada.
2 According to Donnel B. Stern (2010), "an interpersonalization" of dissociation occurs in the analytic intersubjective field. That is, the analyst enacts what the patient dissociates, and the patient enacts what the analyst dissociates. This enactment is surmounted only when either party can attain a reflective perch in their own mind from which to observe this dynamic.
3 Subsequent to my first presentation of this material in 2005, Hazel Ipp and Malcom Slavin (Ipp, 2016) coined the term "complex, achieved empathy." They are delineating

a particularly relational form of empathy "as evolving over time and contingent upon certain psychic work being achieved through hard-earned and deep processing together that enables the varying self-states of analyst and patient to be held simultaneously . . . . Achieved empathy, as we refer to it, emerges through the process of navigating our way through complex experiences and enactments together that include differing, often conflicting self-states, activated in concert and dissociated in concert" (p. 12).

4 We are both aware that my words have touched him in some way. Naming or inquiring about his tears would shut his process down. As Daniel Stern (2004) writes: "Several of my colleagues have asked why the therapist does not at some point verbally mark such a nodal happening—for instance by saying, 'Something important just happened between us.' The reason is this: the therapist and patient already know that something important has happened. They are still reeling under the force of the event" (p. 170).

   Furthermore, I'm not alone in my belief that certain genuine affects—when left alone—move forward on their own. According to Daniel Stern (2004), "Moving along can lead to sudden, dramatic therapeutic changes by way of 'now moments' and 'moments of meeting.' The intersubjective field can be dramatically reorganized at key moments. This occurs when the current state of implicit relational knowing is sharply thrown into question and basic assumptions about the relationship are placed at stake" (p. 165).

References

Aron, L. (1992). Interpretation as expression of the analyst's subjectivity. *Psychoanalytic Dialogues, 2,* 475–507.

Bromberg, P. (1998). *Standing in the spaces: Essays on clinical process, trauma, and dissociation.* Hillsdale, NJ: The Analytic Press.

Davies, J. M. (1999). Getting cold feet, defining "safe-enough" borders: Dissociation, multiplicity, and integration in the analyst's experience. *Psychoanalytic Quarterly, 68,* 184–208.

Freud, S. (1912). Recommendations to physicians practicing psychoanalysis. *Standard Edition, 12,* 109–120.

Ipp, H. (2016). Interweaving the Symbolic and nonsymbolic in therapeutic action: Discussion of Gianni Nebbiosi's "The Smell of Paper." *Psychoanalytic Dialogues, 26,* 10–16.

McLaughlin, J. T. (1991). Clinical and theoretical aspects of enactment. *Journal of the American Psychoanalytic Association, 39,* 595–614.

Mitchell, S. A. (2000). *Relationality: from attachment to intersubjectivity.* Hillsdale, NJ: The Analytic Press.

Ogden, T. H. (1994). The concept of interpretive action. In T. H. Ogden, *Subjects of analysis* (pp. 107–135) Northvale, NJ: Jason Aronson.

Pizer, B. (1997). When the analyst is ill: Dimensions of self-disclosure. *Psychoanalytic Quarterly, 66,* 450–469.

Solomon, D. (2005). The rescue artist. *The New York Times Magazine,* pp. 40–45.

Stern, D. B. (1997). *Unformulated experience: From dissociation to imagination in psychoanalysis.* Hillsdale, NJ: The Analytic Press.

Stern, D. B. (2010). *Partners in thought; Working with unformulated experience, dissociation, and enactment.* New York, NY: Routledge.

Stern, D. N. (2004). *The present moment in psychotherapy and everyday life.* New York, NY: W.W. Norton & Company.

Chapter 7

From Black Hole to Potential Space

Discussion of Barbara Pizer's "'Eva, Get the Goldfish Bowl': Affect and Intuition in the Analytic Relationship"[1]

Stuart A. Pizer

From the perspective of 2005 when I presented this discussion of "'Eva, Get the Goldfish Bowl': Affect and Intuition in the Analytic Relationship" (Chapter 6), we can appreciate, welcome, even marvel at, and use "Eva" as the latest in a series of contributions beginning with Barbara's 1997 paper on self-disclosure ("When the Analyst Is Ill: Dimensions of Self-Disclosure," Chapter 2); and continuing through her important concept of the "relational (k)not" ("When the Crunch Is a (K)not: A Crimp in Relational Dialogue," Chapter 3); and then to her contribution of the nonanalytic third and the analyst's introduction of poetry, both literally and tonally, into the analytic process ("Passion, Responsibility, and 'Wild Geese': Creating a Context for the Absence of Conscious Intentions," Chapter 4). (And here I offer a disclosure of my own: Barbara Pizer is my wife.)

Barbara's consistent project strikes me as an exploration of how the analyst's personhood, including the analyst's disciplined reflective mindfulness, enters the relationship and process with a creative power. Barbara offers us the dialectic of containment and enlivenment within the analyst's subjectivity as a coconstructor of transformations with and for the patient. Thus, a black hole may become a potential space. In a sense, Barbara's paper presents to us her theory of psychological black holes and how the analytic process may approach them and, just possibly, negotiate the bedeviling paradox of how too much has become nothing. I will say more about this soon.

First, as preparation, I find it interesting to juxtapose Barbara's analytic work at the edge of black holes with her work when she finds herself cinched within a transference-countertransference relational (k)not. This requires an extended quote from Barbara's 2003 paper, "When the Crunch Is a

DOI: 10.4324/9781032666303-9

(K)not: A Crimp in Relational Dialogue." As you read the following, note the resonances with "'Eva, Get the Goldfish Bowl'" that, without repetitiveness, convey the integrity of an analytic sensibility. Quoting Barbara:

> Good therapy or analysis provides a crucible for emotional growth. It puts *both participants* in touch with a pain that they have not felt before, a pain that enables *memory* as opposed to repetition—a lost memory or a memory of loss, loss of what once was or should have been and was not, memories that must be borne and grieved …. For the person sitting in the analyst's place, the capacity to contain and negotiate the treatment process requires, as Russell emphasizes, *involvement*. The analyst's involvement with "who the *patient* is, with who he is as he is with the patient, and with what is now *happening*, most especially between them … takes work. The hardest part is the pain. The pain of memory (p. 215)."
>
> Russell concludes, "The technique I have found, if I can call it that, is to try to know the time and the place where I become uninvolved. The most dangerous part of the treatment process is when both parties wish for, invite, non-involvement. That is the most dangerous repetition (pp. 215–216)."
>
> We might surmise that the noninvolvement Russell describes has to do with the potential consequences of too much affect in the consulting room. I mean here, however, to identify a particular situation … that silently dictates disengagement, a kind of petrified distortion from the past [and here, parenthetically, I think of Julian's rocky overhang, stone relics, and adamant positions] that enters present dialogue and contributes to what I have come to call a relational (k)not …. When the crunch is a (k)not,… a particular crimp in relational dialogue occurs, a negating of space and involvement and therefore a negating of the actual current relationship …. Recognition, acknowledgement, and genuine affect necessarily drop out. Without a true dialogical space in this relationship, internal reflection, the capacity for mentalization, is compromised; the possibilities for negotiation between participants are diminished, knotted up, or nullified." (pp. 35–36, in Chapter 3)

Later in that same paper, Barbara lists the common characteristics and consequences of relational (k)nots:

The (k)not collapses potential space and paradox.

The (k)not is nonnegotiable.

The (k)not challenges/stunts affective development.

The (k)not is a negation of ownership of affect, wish, belief, intention.

The (k)not provides a kind of "grief insurance" that protects itself from the awareness of the pain of memory.

The (k)not is a device that dismantles/disassembles involvement.

And, therefore, (k)nots are repeatedly installed for the purpose of preserving attachments that are felt to be necessary for survival.

(p. 45)

According to Barbara, the technique for loosening the grip of relational (k)nots includes the analyst's risking of elements of her own subjectivity, offered spontaneously and authentically, perhaps taking both parties by surprise—a leap of "other-than-me-substance" that, as Barbara ventures, "may open a space that analytic 'clarification,' 'interpretation,' 'inquiry,' or analytic silence may not provide" (p. 52).

Now informed by Barbara's ideas about the (k)not, let us approach the black hole. Both the (k)not and the black hole negate potential space, but I think they do so very differently. The (k)not collapses paradox through a dissociative and projective-introjective enactment in the analytic moment, as a consequence of which the analyst finds herself trapped in a diminished space, without the mental room to think or the relational room to sustain an inquiring or recognizing dialogue. The analyst finds herself caught in the (k)not.

In contrast, the black hole strikes me as highly paradoxical. It is a place where, for the patient, there is nothing there because too much has been stuffed inside. And the analyst finds herself not caught inside a stifling intersubjective bind, but kept outside of a patient's vast intrasubjective gap, an impenetrable emptiness into which so much has been lost through psychic implosion. Inside a (k)not, the analyst's dilemma is "How can I get out so that I may again introduce to you something separate to engage dialogue?" At the edge of a black hole, the analyst's dilemma is "How can I get in, to a place that has not yet come into existence, so that I can offer to the voided density within you a chance to emerge into experience and potential dialogue?"

I do not claim to understand black holes as they are interpreted in theoretical physics. But I gather from Julian that much controversy has surrounded the question of whether inside black holes there exists nothing (as Hawking hypothesizes) or, essentially, more than can fit inside. The latter theory would hold, I believe, that so much matter has concentrated powerfully into the creation of a black hole, perhaps through a collapsing star, that its implosive force is greater than the speed of light. So that even light cannot get out because it, of course, cannot travel faster than the speed of light. According to this alternative theory, one that Julian seems currently to favor, there is nothing in a black hole because there is no way out (at least, not without some transformations in the nature of the matter, the content, if any exists). My mind boggles at this paradox.

I take comfort in turning to psychoanalytic conceptualizing and to Barbara's psychological black-hole theory. What I am calling Barbara's black-hole theory is a particularly relational metaphor for the unconscious. A black hole contains more than you can fit and articulate within the continuity of the developing mind. It represents, by being unrepresentable, overwhelm stored inside subjectivity, the derivative of the trauma of experiencing and *feeling* far too much in the absence of relational containment, acceptance, or recognition. So, instead, what results within the person is an implosive containment, managed through control (and let's note Julian's control!). In the mind's black hole there is nothing there, because it's all *so* there that nothing can be articulated into distinct existence. Where no relational release or bridge has existed to connect inside and outside, no potential space has opened for the negotiation of meaningful experience.

Barbara, typical of her courageous writing that accounts for herself in the analytic intersubjective equation, describes her own "go[ing]-dumb" state (p. 91). Surely more circumscribed than Julian's, Barbara's going-dumb state—described as "boundless, a sucking down"—may be in its own way an intrapsychic black hole, where *too much* experience and more affect than could be delineated, mentalized, or formulated in her developmental ecosystem becomes the "no content" that is the derivative of unmetabolizable content. Going dumb is Barbara's experience of a black hole inside—as if, while in that state, nothing is there, and nothing can get out into words. Barbara now tells us this is "the outcome of whatever seemed to me so present in that dining room but never spoken" (p. 93).

What a compelling image for the origin of intrapsychic black holes: the unspeakable. Perhaps we should remember to bear in mind as we reenter our consulting rooms that "Nothing" may signal "Too much!" Perhaps for Barbara there remains a place where there is still too much to articulate, a place that continues to hold the belief that her passing her chemistry regents is a testament to sister Ilse's fortitude. I ask Barbara, may it also be a testament to whatever else you continue to leave out of the equation in the context of a selectively absent potential space for your articulation of so much?

As analyst, Barbara seeks to locate a potential space for the contents of Julian's black hole to come into existence. Which brings us to Barbara's subtitle: "Affect and Intuition in the Analytic Relationship." Barbara, like Paul Russell (2006), places at the forefront the importance of affective competence, our ability to render our charged experience into words rather than petrified or adamant repetitions. Is the repetition compulsion a black hole into which the present relational moment is drawn and cannot emerge intelligibly? How is the black hole related to Donnel B. Stern's (1997) notion of an unformulated unconscious? Or Bollas' (1987) idea of moods as conveyers of the unthought known, the details of family life enshrouded in a moody fog state? Certainly, the black hole reminds me of what I (1998) meant in writing that all deep analytic work occurs at the edge of the non-negotiable. But how to negotiate the emergence of whatever is in a black hole into the symbolizing realm of potential space?

Barbara's answer is both brand new and paradoxically as old as psychoanalytic thinking. She commends to us what she calls the "outrageous interpretation." By braiding intellect and affect, and also the intersubjective resonances of self and other, she throws a rope into the black hole. We word ourselves out of the black hole of our isolation. And finding the words is a relational process, a negotiation of meanings that is both expression and containment at the same time. Our loneliness is the black hole of experience that we cannot share because we were never recognized. And as a consequence, such experience remains unrepresented verbally in our mind, leaving an empty space. Reading Barbara's paper, I kept thinking of the title of Marie Cardinal's (1983) book *The Words to Say It*. With the words to say it, much like Freud's notion of hypercathexis, there is movement from unconscious primary process to preconscious secondary process, but not out of a dynamic unconscious! Rather, in Barbara's implicit model, affectively charged words sponsor movement out of a relationally nullified unconscious that has been left with experience that remains unformulatable—like the patient who once said to me that there was a special meaning to him in the box-top message "Void Where Prohibited."

Barbara's "outrageous interpretation" reminds me of Strachey's (1934) recommendation to interpret at the moment of affective ripeness, but with a vital difference. How, after all, are we to reach the affectively intense moment in the analytic process when it remains perpetually voided inside a patient's black hole? What Barbara adds here is that the analyst may introduce affect as a way to grab onto, hold, and move affect forward. I have written elsewhere (1998, 2008, 2014, 2022) about the analyst's functions of containment, acceptance, and recognition in the face of the nonnegotiable. Barbara clearly offers Julian a containment profoundly missing from his effaced, grieving, preoccupied, and misrecognizing mother and his ebullient but self-absorbed father. She empathically accepts his rigidity, his rules, without prematurely challenging his part in an ossified marriage. But her recognition is what strikes me as so powerful because, melding her intuitive registration of Julian with her tacit recognition of herself in Julian, Barbara startles them both with powerfully enacted moments of recognition that happen so fast that they may just exceed the speed of light necessary to engage the affective life held within the black hole. As Barbara puts it in her key statement on "technique"—the outrageous method in her madness—"My efforts were focused on an attempt to connect a heretofore dissociated space with affective energy" (p. 102). Thus Barbara moves affect forward.

I wryly conjecture that Barbara's father had his own raw talent for outrageous interpretation. His "Eva, get the goldfish bowl" strikes me as an act of containment that, while it had mockery in it, also came from a loving place. Even if Barbara's father was seeking to control her affect, with its own unfortunate results, his remark differs from the kind of nonrecognition that induces black holes because he was at least meeting intensity with intensity. I suggest that his quip was far more containing than the silences that left Julian alone with his intense and intensely hot core. Was Barbara's first outrageous intervention her own version of "Eva, get the goldfish bowl"—that is, a recognition that reaches deep, touches, and paradoxically contains by startling?

I feel like I've only just started this discussion, but the constraints of space are my container here. So, I will share some more ideas, briefly, in the form of bullet points.

Are Barbara and Julian both rescuers who recognize this dimension in each other? And do they also have in common that they were both wise, old beyond their age when young; and now, in adulthood, younger than their age? What a vulnerable and outrageous little girl this mature analyst can so effectively be. And Julian, skipping three grades, doing his internationally famed work while dressed as a youthful boy, conjuring in his Dream Scene 4 the sparkling pixie dust of Peter Pan.

And does Julian sense with Barbara that these two rescuers also have in common that they were the family "delinquents," the troublemakers whose outrageous actions, like the Winnicottian antisocial gesture, constituted a reaching out with waving arms for intervention, containment, recognition, a meeting of energy with a reassuringly matching energy? And might this mutual intuiting be one of their important intersubjective connectors?

Was Julian's rigid and adamant requirement that Carrie have four children his own rocky overhang imposed as a repetition on his wife? Is there a telescoping of generations in Julian's family life whereby it is assumed that the child repairs a broken marriage? Do we hear Julian perpetuating this with his own forms of unreflective and unrecognizing love? In fantasy, is Julian, the rescuer, reparatively making babies with his mother and, thus, in his own intersubjective way shaping the Carrie he's faced with, identified with, and unable to see as separate?

Similarly, when Julian followed the post-op instructions "to a tee" was his adamant self looking scientifically at the instructions more than he looked recognizingly at Carrie? Is this a legacy of his own history of not being recognized as well as their marital history? Was it the flexible or the adamant part of Julian that was doing the tending? Does this come into question during a period of analytic containment and acceptance?

In Barbara's response to Julian's harshness with his eldest daughter—in her quick switch from "not too good" to "but on the other hand" (p. 100) — is she saying that Julian's harsh house rules are containing for his daughter, grounding for her adolescent angst? Is it a legacy of "Eva, get the goldfish bowl" that Barbara is ready to see the good, perhaps the reassurance, in forms of paternal toughness?

Does Julian's piercingly certain reaction to Barbara's "crossing the line" by giving him her paper carry, in part, his jealousy of the patient Sam so extensively described in that paper? Julian contends that Barbara is looking for his care. Could it be that Julian can read in Barbara's paper what an amazing caregiver she is and might he wonder if her caregiving may be driven by an urgency born of her own unrecognized needs? And indeed, the urgency of unrecognized needs may be a vulnerability in all of us who have become caregivers while relegating aspects of our attachment system into necessarily dissociated black holes. Does Julian's protest include the glimmerings of explicit intersubjective recognition in the analytic relationship, or a last-ditch effort on Julian's part to fight against opening to love, opening beyond what Barbara so incisively calls his narrowed vision, and allowing himself to be, to be with, to allow the sting of memory, grief, and entry into relatedness?

Finally, a response to Barbara's ending thoughts about our liability to falling into the well of our own loneliness. Can the caregiver's own needs ever be faced? And do they have a place in the therapeutic relationship? I circle back to the beginning of Barbara's paper, where she quotes the rescue artist, Johnathan Foer, "'I write because I want to end my loneliness' (p. 43)" (p. 89). I recall that between college years filled with Shakespeare and Saul Bellow and volunteering at a state mental hospital, I had a summer job writing for *The New Yorker* under the tutelage of William Shawn. What could be more fulfilling, more precociously culminating, than the prospect of graduating from college to begin as a staff writer for "Talk of the Town"? But instead, at the end of my second summer there, I told Mr. Shawn that I'd decided to become a psychotherapist. Sitting alone in my New Yorker office, finding publishable words that did not arise from my own black holes, I recognized that I needed my life's work to be in an office with someone else there. What a privilege to be present with and for others, to become an agent of presence in an enlivened relational field.

I'll conclude with a quote from James McLaughlin (1995), dear to both Barbara and me:

> The course of any analysis can be described as a mutual exploring of the communicative boundaries of one by the other in the intimacy of the analytic dyad, with the aim of both to reach the core of the other while protecting one's own, and to avoid suffering its opposite.

> And what each of us needs from the other, whether on the couch or behind it, is at depth pretty much the same. We need to find in the other an affirming witness to the best that we hope we are, as well as an accepting and durable participant to those worst aspects of ourself that we fear we are. We seek to test ourself in the intimacy of the therapeutic relationship, to have what we are become known to and accepted by the other, in whose sum we may more fully accept ourself. (p. 434)

Like Barbara, I prefer the containment of the goldfish bowl to a prematurely Buddhist "no self" solo on the mountain, a black hole on a rocky ledge.

Note

1 An earlier version of this discussion was presented on May 14, 2005, for an invited program at the Toronto Institute for Contemporary Psychoanalysis, Toronto, Canada.

References

Bollas, C. (1987). *The shadow of the object: Psychoanalysis of the unthought known*. New York, NY: Columbia University Press.

Cardinal, M. (1983). *The words to say it*. New York: Van Vactor & Goodheart.

McLaughlin, J. T. (1995). Touching limits in the analytic dyad. *Psychoanalytic Quarterly*, *LXIV*, 433–465.

Pizer, S. A. (1998). *Building bridges: The negotiation of paradox in psychoanalysis*. Hillsdale, NJ: The Analytic Press.

Pizer, S. A. (2008). The shock of recognition: What my grandfather taught me about psychoanalytic process. *International Journal of Psychoanalytic Self Psychology*, *3*, 287–303.

Pizer, S. A. (2014). The analyst's generous involvement. *Psychoanalytic Dialogues*, *24*, 1–13.

Pizer, S. A. (2022). *Building bridges: The negotiation of paradox in psychoanalysis*. Classic Edition. New York, NY: Routledge.

Russell, P. L. (2006). Trauma, repetition, and affect. *Contemporary Psychoanalysis*, *42*, 601–636.

Stern, D. B. (1997). *Unformulated experience: From dissociation to imagination in psychoanalysis*. Hillsdale, NJ: The Analytic Press.

Strachey, J. (1934). The nature of the therapeutic action of psychoanalysis. *International Journal of Psychoanalysis*, *15*, 127–159.

Reverie

A Motherless Child

Deep inside the night, I lie in my bed and listen for the whistle of a distant train echoing through the darkness. And then the melody comes back to me. I hear it through, a couple times, before I get the words.

   Sometimes I feel like a motherless child,

   Sometimes I feel like a motherless child,

   Sometimes I feel like motherless child,

   A long way from home.

It's the melody that haunts me—not the words. The words don't have to do with me. I love my mother very much.

Besides which, she lives in the same town.

DOI: 10.4324/9781032666303-10

Chapter 8

Risk and Potential in Analytic Disclosure

Can the Analyst Make "the Wrong Thing" Right?

After completing a brief intensive five-month treatment of somebody else's patient–the first breaking of the frame–and worrying if the analyst can make the "wrong thing right" (Levenon, 2000), I discovered Levenson's remark on the work of Warren Poland:

> Poland's very attempts at grasping his own participation and formalizing it as a clinical technique ... could paradoxically work to his disadvantage. ... [I]t has long been common knowledge that atypical interventions seem to work best when they are both spontaneous and contrary to the therapist's sense of appropriate technique. That is, the intervention only works when it is the *wrong* thing to do. Once it is sanitized, legitimized, sanctified as appropriate technique, it falls flat. (p. 68)

What's my story then? If we agree that "wrong" interventions may "work" only when they are not replicated, or sanctified in terms of "appropriate technique," what am I talking about? What purpose does this narrative serve? I venture to say that whereas spontaneous interventions may be nontransportable, the principles that guide the choices we make *or alter* in relation to what we hold as essential to "appropriate practice" must have some general application that can, indeed, be considered. Thus, to consider whether any analyst has the power or the right to make the wrong thing right, in this particular case, including the paradoxical risks and potentials in an act of disclosure, it becomes important to know where the analyst is coming from: that is, what matrix of abiding principles guides her sense of "appropriate technique" in the clinical moment?

So here's my story.

DOI: 10.4324/9781032666303-11

The Analyst's Personal Legacy

Issues involving disclosure and confidentiality are bred in my bones. My mother was so private about her person that I grew up knowing as much about her feelings as I knew about the mailman or a neighbor next door. I saw her cry only twice in my young life: once when she caught me, at the age of ten, with stolen money in my pocket, and then again in a rare instance when I heard my father raise his voice to her. My older sister, Ilse, and I were sitting at the breakfast table, and my father's face turned black as he actually *forbade* my mother to go alone to Brooklyn to visit her older brother, who had come in from South America. Ilse, appalled by this sound and sight, fled the room. I, on the other hand, stayed put, screaming at Dad for mistreating my mother. He must have appreciated that in principle because for once he didn't "command respect" and tell me to "control myself." "Respect your elders" (particularly applied to me in the familiar form of "No back talk, Barbara!") and "Children should be seen and not heard" were among the general principles bestowed on kids who were stuck with parents from the old country.

My parents were refugees who came here just before World War II. My Dad, a Jew and a doctor of law in Germany, decided to leave with his wife and one-year-old daughter, despite his family's objections. (They were convinced that this Hitler thing would "blow over.") Dad, at thirty-two, landed a job as a messenger boy, which earned him enough to go back to night school for an American law degree, thus leaving his wife and daughter, Ilse, (I would be born—a preemie—eight months later) to fend largely for themselves in this strange land. Nevertheless, throughout my growing up, I hardly ever saw my mother cry. Not even as we sat in the waiting room at The Massachusetts General Hospital where she, still beautiful to me in her eighties, and I—a seasoned psychologist—awaited the examinations she insisted on in order to determine whether or not she had Alzheimer's disease. I picture my mother now, leaning back in the chair next to me and closing her eyes.

And then, with no preamble whatsoever, she said, "Barbara, did you know that I was sexually abused by my older brother?"

"*What?*" I couldn't believe my ears.

"From the ages of five … or maybe seven to nine."

"What happened?"

"My parents sent him away. Eventually he went to South America."

I can still hear myself responding, in a long-forgotten voice: "Have you told Daddy this?"

"Yes," she said, "last week."

"Last week?"

"Your father always had a funny feeling about my brother. Never trusted him."

Dad, though more expressive than my mother, was an old-fashioned lawyer through and through. Although he would spend many a dinner conversation—in the spirit of furthering his children's education—putting before us the problems presented by legal cases he was dealing with, the cases were always disguised and peopled by fictional names. He was adamant about issues of ethics, including matters involving confidentiality. For example, when he discovered that my sister finally "tattled on me" for having committed an infraction because I wouldn't continue to scratch her back whenever she wanted me to, the punishment for my bad behavior was suddenly suspended, and we had to sit down and listen to a lengthy lecture on the evils of "blackmail." In his later years, my father, with great regret, told us that he never imagined that he would grow old enough to be ashamed of his profession. Whereas mother's affectionate phrase for the man she married was "an overgrown boy scout," my image of myself was that of a lawyer's daughter who also carried the legacy of her mother's humiliating pain. Matters of disclosure were matters of great moment, as were issues of trust and confidentiality.

The Analyst and Her Patient: A Theoretical Statement

So the story of an illustrative treatment begins with my own disclosures. I realize full well that this sort of focus presents a ready invitation to those disapproving critics who claim that relational analysts spend far too much time and energy talking about themselves and their own processes at the expense of what's going on inside the patient. Such an argument, of course, presupposes a unidirectional economy. But if we can agree that there are at least two people in the consulting room, that existing within each of these people are multiple self-states brought to life in intersubjectively evocative interactions, then there can be no analysis of the person in the patient's place without concurrent scrutiny of what's going on inside the person sitting in the analyst's place, and how she may be contributing to whatever occurs in the moment. Nobody says it is easy, or even fully possible, but that is the relational effort.

To my mind, a major defining feature of an analytic process has more to do with how we use ourselves—with developing the ability to analyze what's happening with those feelings and figures (past and present) that people use in our attempts at healing work with others— than with the "use of the couch" or the number of times a week, or one particular theory, or the specific nature of "the frame." What can we really "know" about another person's psyche, other than what we, ourselves, imagine from the questions that we think to ask, the hunches that develop from past experience, and the intersubjective present interaction? All we have to offer is our listening presence, along with some tentative speculations whose signals must first originate from our own personal data bank. But where and how does analytic disclosure fit in our definition of what we call "the analytic frame"?

Contrary to a common myth, analytic disclosure is not what relational theory or technique is all about. To assume as much would be like saying that baking powder is the ingredient that constitutes a particular cake, or knowing how to steer a car defines a good driver. Although disclosure of one sort or another is certainly one consequence of any intimate analytic engagement, it is far from the central feature of relational "technique." Whatever our individual differences, and without ignoring the asymmetrical roles between analyst and patient, relationalists take into account the mutual influence that two people have on one another (see Aron, 1992).

From this perspective, the analytic pair negotiates a "frame" that allows potential space—for the person in the patient's place as well as the person in the analyst's place—to emerge freely, while simultaneously preserving and still maintaining the basic integrity and necessary privacy required by each party in the dyad. That is quite a mouthful. And of course, as analysts we know that we will fall short of this ideal. In the best of times we may succeed and we have to fail. The frame, in my mind, is never "fixed," but consists of an amalgam of the particular "given circumstances" unique to the participants in each analytic dyad. The frame, in my view, like the requirements of a sonnet's construction, is a needed container that permits a maximum of intimate freedom (see B. Pizer, 2003). So once again we might ask, can the analyst make the wrong thing right?

Case Vignette

Actually, the vignette I relate comes from the brief treatment between Kate and myself that begins with a broken frame. I had gotten to know her in another context. I supervised her for two years, beginning in 1988. At that time, she came recommended to me by her colleagues. She was also recommended by Ariel, her therapist, whom I had once known well, and to whom I felt deeply attached, even though—given life's circumstances—I had not spent time with her for more than a decade. In the course of supervision with Kate, a gifted clinician herself, working with deeply disturbed patients, I came to learn of her own traumatic past, which included severe neglect, sexual abuse, repeated abandonment, and ultimately a hospitalization that could have been averted under better circumstances. In those days, the hospital served as fertile breeding ground for further traumatizations, and in this latest context, Kate felt finally "rescued" by Ariel.

That would have been about fourteen years prior to the Monday morning in February 2002 when Kate called me, frantic. Ariel, after careful preparation with Kate around a routine day surgery on the previous Friday—and as a way of assuring Kate of her sense of certainty that she would come through fine—promised to listen to the phone messages that Kate could leave on her machine over the weekend. Also, she assured Kate she would reply before their appointment on the following Monday afternoon. Indeed, Kate did leave messages on Ariel's machine. A dissociated memory from childhood jarred her awake that night, a vivid rendering so filled with terror and compliance that she knew it would disintegrate and therefore asked that Ariel save the scene on tape for when they met, so they could tackle it together.

But not a word from Ariel. *No word at all* until that Monday morning when she received "this weird sounding message" from Ariel's husband. It said that Ariel had contracted "the flu" and would be "out" for the rest of the week. Something sounded fishy ... unreal ... and certainly unlike Ariel. For more than fourteen years, until this day, Ariel had never denied Kate access, or gone back on what Kate had considered "her word." The frame they created over fourteen years included regular phone contact, and today this frame had not simply been broken, it was shattered, and I could feel its fragments vibrating through the wires—fragments that I felt were now bequeathed to me.

"Something's happened," Kate whispered, "I need you to find out what's happened. Please Barbara, *I need your help!*"

Just ten minutes before my first patient of the morning would arrive. The space that emergency inflicts on time is paradoxical. There is an experience of slow motion as one moves about in a context of fast-forward events outside of human control. Quickly I ascertained from Ariel's distraught husband how she had, as predicted, undergone the surgery without a glitch. The thing happened in the recovery room. Suddenly Ariel could no longer speak. Cerebral hemorrhage—euphemism for a stroke. Etiology unknown. Prognosis uncertain. Ariel incommunicado.

"Please Barbara, I need your help!"

Even though our supervisory relationship had terminated two years earlier, and even though I had not crossed paths with her therapist for many years before that, I had become aware from the way we had worked together—weathering the difficulties with her and her patients—that I had earned a rare place near Ariel in the narrow arena of Kate's sense of trust.

"Please Barbara ... "

I tell my supervisees that the concept of soul saving is anathema to the work of therapy and that therapists who believe in sacrifice for the sake of their patients end up punishing both parties. Furthermore, if I were asked to take a supervisee in treatment I would most certainly decline. In this very moment, however, I found myself in a unique position between Ariel and Kate—and for reasons I could not explain—somehow automatically responsible to do the best I could for Kate. We arranged a time to talk.

I told Kate that given the ambiguity and constraints already built into our situation, the limits of both our schedules, I would make every attempt to try and see her twice a week until we could know more about what the future held. I would charge her for the time. My goal would be to hold, bear, normalize, and put into perspective Kate's experiencing of Ariel's absence in its ongoing context. My role would be similar to that of a covering clinician, but in addition I would keep Kate informed of Ariel's current condition so far as I could know it. And so we began our work.

Piece by piece, over the coming months, Kate and I would negotiate our own peculiar working frame that altered shape with the slightest change in our environment: news of improvement or setback in Ariel's condition, the threat of a simple head cold in either one of us, the shock of learning that the tape on which Kate had deposited her traumatic memories had been erased, a miscommunication between the two of us. Any of these occurrences were either heralded or followed by a new, more frightening set of dissociations. And we couldn't tell whose psyche triggered them or what came first, external event or internal chaos. In each of these situations, I would try to follow Kate's lead, with one terrible exception. But before reporting fragments from this vignette, I need to double back for the sake of orientation.

From February through June, Kate and I moved from enactment through enactment, wending our uncertain way in a recursive series of little moments of trauma and recovery, rupture and repair, as we constructed new experience with tools that were often unfamiliar to us both. For example, Ariel's dear friend Corey became the third party in our process, the go-between who kept me regularly informed of Ariel's condition and prognosis. With Ariel's permission, Kate and I agreed to my disclosures of these conversations in order to provide enough information to relay a clear picture of how Ariel was doing. That strategy seemed right to us, particularly in view of Kate's crazy, drunken mother whom Kate had always taken care of and who would consistently deny her little girl's query with the comment, "Don't be silly, Katie, that's not vomit that you smell in the kitchen, I am *cleaning* the sink." But soon after we learned that Ariel was well enough to leave the hospital and enter rehab, Kate's relief quickly transformed to rage over Ariel's abandonment and led her to instruct me otherwise. "I don't want to hear another word about what's going on with her, unless it's dire; my anger makes me feel too crazy."

This change in Corey's function and Kate's request for my withholding, provided me a new awareness of our threesome, as well as an important clue about dyads and triads that I would pick up later.

Throughout this treatment, as Ariel relearned to speak, had visitors, gradually began her preparations for return to work, I had sadly come to recognize that I would have to forgo my impulse for direct communication with her. Despite a heightening desire to visit with Ariel, to see her with my own eyes and in this act to comfort both of us who had meant so much to one another in another time, to talk with her directly about our mutual charge, it became clear that the most loving thing to do was continue contact through her intermediary. Now my first allegiance was to my current patient, Kate, and it became increasingly imperative for me to stay as close as possible to her experience of cutoff.

The Moment of Truth

Here I introduce the vignette with excerpts from Kate's phone messages now received on *my* machine. I have asked her to try and flush out more words for the feeling she calls "scared," to find the fine distinctions between angry, sad, and scared, to locate the exact triggers and tell me where the feelings are directed—toward me, toward Ariel, toward herself.

"What do I mean right now by feeling scared. Being depressed. Being alone and not wanting to talk to anybody...Not mattering to anybody. When I'm getting more depressed, I get really scared about that. If I ever have to go back to the hospital, it will kill me I know."

"I'm fried. This case I'm working on is triggering me up the ying-yang! I feel really scared. Traumatized. A million different things. I don't want to do this anymore. I'm enraged. I guess I'm scared about coming in tomorrow, fearful about what's going to happen when it starts coming out ..."

Kate is weeping as she enters my office. The loss of her recovered memories that somebody erased from Ariel's machine enrages her. Who would dare to touch them, erase them? Furthermore, they have come back.

Furthermore, she never told me how, on that weekend of Ariel's surgery, when she didn't hear a word in reply, she walked out on the sixth-floor ledge of a building, and sat there until she frightened herself back in.

"I knew it. I knew it wouldn't be all right. She heard my messages and never called me back. I knew ..."

As the words tumble out, I watch her disappear—dissociate and shatter. Hard as I try, I cannot reach the blank white Kate. Gone. *Where is Ariel now when we need her*? The vibrating fragmentation in the room, an electrifying echo of crickets in my ears, becomes more than I can bear. I experience a visceral fear for whatever may be left of a life. Heart in mouth, I do something I have never done before or ever wish to do again. I say that in spite of current circumstances, there is *in fact* an underlying continuity containing us here. And now is the time to speak out loud about it.

I say to Kate that way back in the seventies, when Ariel was still a psychology student in training, we were engaged in a process similar to the process that she has been engaged in with Ariel. (Ariel was my analysand.) I say that when Kate sits with me, we *both* carry Ariel inside. Along with all the pain that all three of us must feel about this break in real time, there exists an awe-inspiring symmetry and continuity that we *can* appreciate. It keeps us all together. Kate does seem to reconstitute on hearing this. The content of my words, I later learn, will get dissociated, but in the moment I ask her how she feels about hearing this. "Good," she tells me, and then as if she's speaking to herself, "makes me feel very good." Even though she leaves my office having come together, I know that this reprieve is temporary. There is so much work to do. But this day gives us time to breathe.

Here we reached a marker moment in our efforts to make some meaning of a strange accident that threw the three of us into unforeseen contact. One is tempted to elaborate our story in greater detail, or bring it to conclusion, if such a thing were possible, but this much serves to raise the question in vivid particular: what are the risks and potentials in analytic disclosure, and can the analyst make the "wrong thing" right?

Even though Kate and Ariel, now engaged together again in a deeper analytic process, express their gratitude, continuing to assure me I have done them no harm, I still continue to wrestle with these questions. Having made my peace with the necessary risks involved in disclosures in general, the more difficult concept for me (a lawyer's daughter) is that of disclosure that interrupts the sanctity of confidentiality. The idea of revealing information about another without express permission remains anathema to me. Of course I do take into consideration (and perhaps find comfort in) Levenson's (2000) further words in that paper from which I have already quoted. Levenson writes, "We are confronted with the possibility that change may take place in those moments when we 'let go' out of despair or fatigue, allowing the patient the necessary room to change autonomously, neither to oppose or submit to us" (p. 68).

But I can see now, after this writing, that doing "the wrong thing" and "letting go" are far from a "free fall." One needs some structure to fall back on. I associate to the memory of myself as a child at the dining room table, screaming at Dad for "mistreating" my mother. "Right" or "wrong," he must have appreciated my "letting go" in principle because for once he didn't command the usual respect and tell me to "control myself." Notions about a hierarchy of essential principles are bred in my bones.

References

Aron, L. (1992). Interpretation as expression of the analyst's subjectivity. *Psychoanalytic Dialogues*, *2*, 475–507.

Levenson, E. (2000). Commentary on Poland, W., Witnessing and otherness. *Journal of the American Psychoanalytic Association*, *1*, 66–71.

Pizer, B. (2003). Reply to commentary of P. Ringstrom on When the crunch is a (k)not. *Psychoanalytic Dialogues*, *13*, 207–210.

Reverie

I Wish That Life

I wish that life would once more lead me through
Sweet memory's gate and take me back to where
I found my senses at the sight of you.
Your focused gaze that felt so hard to bear
Reminded me of unknown broken ties
The way you took me in and held me there
As if I'd fallen *up* into your eyes!
Oh how enchantment tricks, and lovers dare
To dance their jigs and play with age and time
So one will suckle while the other nurse
Until sensations rise and turn sublime
And I cry out, for we are both immersed.
It's not that Love o'ertakes or tears apart,
But makes me more *myself*, and breathing from the heart.

DOI: 10.4324/9781032666303-12

Chapter 9

The Heart of the Matter in Matters of the Heart

Power and Intimacy in Analytic and Couples Relationships[1]

Introduction

Stuart and I have been together for fifty years. According to some of our closest friends, we "come as a set." Not to say that we do not heartily disagree at times—with a passionate intensity that leads us ultimately to understand one another even more deeply. Despite our individual ways and clinical practices, we often work as couple cotherapists and coteachers. At a recent clinical seminar, we were asked how each of us might respond to a particular stuck moment in an already sticky situation with a patient. Toward the end of the seminar, a participant remarked, "I'm not exactly sure of how to put this, but there's much more to get from what you've said than what you've said." She tried to shake the bewildering recognition off with a flicking of her hands. "Your hypothetical interventions are so completely different.... Even though they get down to the same intent, they evolve from different conceptual places. And so it's hard to get my head around the fact that both of them feel right."

Thus, in the spirit of such a partnership, I am indeed pleased to continue on from where Stuart left off in his 2008 article, "The Shock of Recognition," an article whose ideas about the transformative power of intimacy in the analytic situation are so poignantly inspired by the remarkable relationship with his beloved stepgrandfather. I certainly concur with Stuart's perspective here and, although I never met Grandpa, I consider myself a sort of third-generation beneficiary of his generosity. What I mean is, Stuart's song-title conclusion in Grandpa's idiom that "You're Nobody 'Til Somebody Loves You" is without question the experience I received through Stuart when he was in graduate school and we first met.

Back then it was Stuart who convinced me that I had what it took to go for a doctorate degree; who listened with an empathic and sponsoring ear

DOI: 10.4324/9781032666303-13

to my groping, self-conscious thoughts and gathered them up into a coherence that I could recognize as my own; who pushed me to word my feelings into communicable form; and who taught me how to write transitions. It was Stuart, undoubtedly influenced by his grandfather's abiding *presence*, who waited beyond all reasonable patience for me to see my way clear to marrying him. In this phase of our being together, as is perhaps common in the first blush of most romances, the intersubjective qualities that Stuart outlines—containment, acceptance, and recognition—were at their peak.

However, when love deepens to the point where two people commit to a lifelong partnership, those qualities of containment, acceptance, recognition, and the quality of presence will necessarily alter over time if the relationship is to grow. What I want to emphasize here is that the emergent landscape in which the transformative power of joint intimacy may flourish in a couple relationship bears less resemblance to that similarly awesome laying down of groundwork and its subsequent unfolding in a caretaking or analytic relationship.

Therefore, it is my intention to explore further the power of intimacy in the context of the consulting room and compare it with an analogous process in a personally committed life partnership.

The distinctions, I believe—quite apart from individual convictions concerning the degree of mutuality in both contexts—begin in the accepted asymmetry of role relationship in the caretaking or analytic dyad. It is interesting to contrast this reality with what goes on between members of a couple. It is not unusual to discover that in the effort to forge a companionship of equals, both partners assiduously collude to deny ownership of personal power. How do power and intimacy go together? I close my introduction with a general proposal.

I propose that in any two-person relationship, analytic or otherwise, the power of intimacy at its best is achieved when there exists a relative balance—acceptable to both participants—in the inevitable dialectic between intimacy and power, a dialectic that cannot remain static and therefore requires mutual awareness and tending from moment to moment.

Intimacy and Power as an Ongoing Dialectic

Taken separately, each of these two terms, *power* and *intimacy*, are loaded with a variety of ill-defined and unspoken meanings—running the entire gamut of what we call "for better or for worse."

In his article "Clinical and Theoretical Aspects of Enactment," McLaughlin (1991) elegantly summarized the issues raised by the power of intimacy taking place behind the consulting room's closed doors:

> Given the potential for regression in both parties induced by the deprivations inherent in the analytic situation, it is expectable that words, as the word "enactment" itself informs us, become acts, things—sticks and stones, hugs and holdings. This secondary process, which we cherish for its linearity and logic, becomes loaded with affective appeal and coercion, [note here the co-presence of expressions suggesting intimacy and power] to be experienced by either or both parties as significant acts or incitement to action. (p. 598)

Note this case in point:[2] Still with some considerable pain and shame, I remember myself as a young intern in the first week of my first analysis. I was so flattered that this particular analyst, highly touted and having somehow reached a kind of guru status among my colleagues, agreed to take me on. I remember confessing to him, as if to a priest, that my excess of trust and expressive nature—although gratifying—had led me to unspeakable troubles. What sort of troubles? A parish priest when I was four years old, a minister-camp counselor when I was ten. Then in a whisper, I heard myself saying, "Seems like I never learned the difference between affection and sexuality. I think I want to be able to express all of my feelings in here without having to worry about its being dangerous to me."

From behind the couch I heard, "I don't promise not to fuck with you."

I remember almost like yesterday, the way my mind sucked in, steadying itself by moving to the *grammar* of the comment. "An odd construction," I thought to myself, trying to unscramble the double negative. Unable to make sense of it, I then focused on the preposition: *with* you? "I don't promise not to fuck you" would be one thing, a bravado argument engaged to send the words away. However, "don't promise not to fuck with you"—what could that mean? Odd. I remember staying silent for a while. I heard the silence in the room. The sound went through me to my toes. Diverting my attention to a different subject, I talked about another thing I cannot now recall.

Some months would pass before the first physical transgression would occur. I do not recall those exact circumstances either, but I know, in the body of my bones, that it all began in the clinical moment when I heard those funny words entering into the back of my head, "I don't promise not to fuck with you."

Stepping outside of the vignette and taking a more reflective view, one can at least imagine how the analyst's unconscious pull toward the taking of power and the seeking of intimacy, as well as the patient's unconscious pull toward surrendering power in exchange for intimacy, predisposes the analytic couple to undermine these essential relational elements. Without containment in his repertoire, the analyst becomes more vulnerable to experiencing such an inner pull in the face of the patient taking, as is her due, the ultimate "credit" for the work; taking, as she must, the analytic gains out of their dyad into the world—thus leaving the analyst who is unable to tolerate acceptance of the patient's individuating dynamics once again abandoned and anonymous in his consulting room. Likewise, without the presence of a containing and accepting analyst, the vulnerable patient must, at some level, experience the wish to gratify the analyst's felt urgency as a repetition of past relationships, as well as her magical wish to have the analytic work of becoming her own person performed for her in exchange for the gift of intimacy.

I believe that from childhood on, most if not all of us have experienced interactions in which a powerful other appears to step down from an anointed perch to that unreal place of promised intimate absolution and, in a charismatic eye-to-eye utterance, instructs: "Trust me." For all of us and for a patient in particular, such a seductive invitation to yield one's own separate locus of power is, without a doubt, a devilish temptation.

Some analysts still maintain that one can avoid the danger of regressive pulls by withdrawal, under the rubric of analytic anonymity and "neutrality," from intimate engagement. Our problem, however, is no longer merely a matter of choice between a classically abstinent or more openly interactive style; we are all of us necessarily cautious and made wary by the unending wave of revelations regarding therapist abuse and subsequent litigations. Here is the dilemma. Strict analytic rules of conduct may protect the analyst and the frame and, as some continue to insist, allow patient and analyst a greater freedom to explore the patient's deepest feelings of anger and desire. But how, actually, is the contemporary patient, no longer schooled in the old medical model of authority, encouraged to take such risks when the analyst minimizes his (see also Mitchell, 2000)?[3]

Now let us construct a dialogical model of both of these terms—power and intimacy—a dialectic defining a range of potential within each term and a scope of possibility between the terms. It seems to me that once we conceptualize power and intimacy as a tension rather than an either-or, we can acknowledge both destructive and constructive aspects in the relationship *between* them as well as *within* them—on each side of that tension.

Destructive power refers to domination, control, defensiveness, competitiveness, and authoritative imposition. Joyce Carol Oates (1993), in an essay on the Deadly Sins, alluded to its underlying motivation when she wrote, "power is, as we know, chiefly concerned with its own preservation." However, if we conceive of power in a tension with intimacy, we are reminded of the constructive or creative power of words; the power entailed in taking or surrendering analytic responsibility; the power of analytic discipline; of the analyst's containment, acceptance, and recognition; and the creative power in the energy drawn from the balance of joint meaning making in the analytic relationship.

Like destructive power, destructive intimacy refers to domination, control, and imposition by seductive means; just as a constructive and balanced intimacy may refer to caring, responsibility, discipline, mutual recognition, shared meaning making, and the experience of a state of awe in the light of new discovery. To my mind, those moments of balance in the dyadic analytic power-intimacy dialectic are those nonverbal moments of mystery where the work seems to move itself forward as the analytic relationship deepens in a way that can neither be fully named nor ever repeated in the same way. Perhaps Stuart would call this "the shock of recognition" in the analytic relationship.

The Shock of Recognition: A Second Vignette

Holding Stuart's (2008) article in mind, let us think—as this next vignette unfolds—how the urgencies for intimacy and power finally arrive at a relatively balanced tension, a state in the consulting room that does require the analyst's disciplined ability to contain and accept what Stuart has called "the nonnegotiable stance of a traumatized patient."

I am lying on the couch, somewhere in the middle of my first year in a second analysis. We are already stuck.[4] "Dr. Silberger," I say, "I don't think you get it. I don't want to be calling *you* by *your* first name. I just would like for you to call *me* by *mine*."

Silence.

"Okay, so what are my associations? They're *not* associations. It feels ridiculous—me telling you these humiliating, intimate details about myself and you responding with 'Well, Dr. Pizer, have you considered' blah blah blah."

From behind the couch, "Why ridiculous?"

"Or you get out of it by not calling me *anything*! I don't know which is worse."

Variations on the theme of this dialogue go on for months. Analytic inquiry yields nothing. For months I cannot seem to relinquish what has grown into an all-out campaign. Despite my best efforts to collaborate, associations all lead back to the present lurch that I feel left in every time I hear myself addressed by my professional title and married name. Silence meets with silence in return. Interpretations of resistance are met with an exhausted sigh, providing only further ammunition that I, in turn, direct back to my accuser.

Then, "It is too often the case," I hear these words make entrance into the back of my head, "that the legacy of trauma in a first analysis is visited upon the second analyst. It sometimes *takes a third treatment to make it right*."

"Well that's just nifty," I sob, "just nifty. First you push me away by refusing me the name I was born with, the name I'm most attached to, the name that means the most to me, the name that I know best … and now you suggest that my honest protest comes from some pathological source that threatens to sabotage our work."

Silence.

"Nifty …" I can hear my voice diminish to a whisper.

This is the mysterious moment in which I recognize that I experience the silence as somehow different. Not between us. What then? Like a silence going on *inside* my analyst. Something like a struggle taking place that he is letting happen. I know that I must wait, and I *want* to wait, and then

"It is clear to me that you would like me to call you by your first name," he said. "But I cannot do it. I cannot do it. It flies in the face of my training. I could not bring myself to do it."

This stunning revelation brings with it a great sense of relief—a transformative moment. Paradoxically, feeling at last intimately met, I am quiet for the rest of the hour.

As Stuart (1998) wrote, "Clearly a counterbalance to a patient's history of misrecognitions, the therapist's recognition in the face of the nonnegotiable is not conveyed through interpretations or explanations, *but only in the form of authentic enactments*" (p. 129, emphasis added).

Dr. Silberger's recognizing revelation contained an acceptance of both his own classical training as well as a resolution of his struggle to accept my nonnegotiable stance without compromising either one of us. Although I surely was not *thinking* about these matters then, I *felt* his presence with me. Hoffman (1998)[5] would have defined Silberger's enactment as "throwing away the book" while maintaining a balance between "analytic discipline and spontaneous expressiveness" or, as I would put it, between power and intimacy. For me, Dr. Silberger's enactment, in which he struggled with an intense loyalty conflict between "the book" he was trained by and a personal commitment to "I-Thou" relating, marked the opening of a critical transformative process in "being" between us.

Over the next several years, I would come to realize, deeply, that intimacy in a partnership (analytic or otherwise) need not require blind conformity. Two people may disagree and differ without catastrophic or lasting rupture. Self-assertion need not be sacrificed at the altar of being with another; one need not be required to sit in the lap of another's outlook on the world to gain respect and care. Furthermore, as Susan Coates (1998) wrote:

> a true meeting of minds requires a small mis-meeting of the minds if the patient is to be recognized and … met. It is this slight mis-meeting that allows a symbolic stance to occur and provides the "creative spark." (p. 128)

Recognition of another in any context does not necessarily imply consensus. As a matter of fact, the closer we come to a "blending" of minds, the further away we get from two-person relating. The transformative power of intimacy from a relational point of view describes a dialectic between and within two subjectivities, between and within power and intimacy as experienced by these two subjectivities.

It seems relevant to note that at the end of my analysis, Dr. Silberger asked if I would agree that we now call each other by our first names, Jay and Barbara. I was touched by his rationale. Because we were both in the field, and would most surely be addressing one another in public, he saw the use of the familiar as a way of *preserving* the intimacy of the relationship we were now terminating.

As final evidence of the lasting transformation marked by my second analyst's enactment, I must admit that the shock of his recognition has transformed itself in current memory. More than ten years after his death, I can still hear the exacting echo of his exasperated phrasings entering my brain: "It is clear to me that you would like me to call you by your first name, Barbara. But I *can not* do it. I *can not* do it."

Blind, Deaf, and Crippled: The Power of Intimacy in Couple Relationships

Naturally in couple relationships, enactments prevail, while explorations that even ever-so-slightly smack of one person's interpretation of another's behavior run the risk of a one-up/one-down power play where usually, understandably, there is hell to pay! Although transference and regression run rampant in romance, what do we do when the blush wears off, when what seemed so wonderful falls flat, and what felt so fresh and tasted so good goes stale? How do two people *talk* about the boredom and the disappointment? Most important of all, when two people are both in need at the *same time*, what happens to containment, acceptance, and recognition? Can there be such a thing as sustained moments of balance between intimacy and power?

In the majority of couples, as I have said, I believe that power is largely denied from the get-go. Power, when conceived as a contradiction of love, gets sneaky and goes underground. For example, when one person experiences vulnerability in conjunction with shame, a functional response goes AWOL, a striking inability to pause reflectively takes over, and present whereabouts are turned around along with the history and reality of current partnership. In this too-familiar danger zone, affects can morph into powerful retreats, disdainful teasing, or all-out aggressive emotional strikes.

On the other hand, Stuart and I have sat with many a couple where the fear of abandonment and well-worn habits of mind wield greater power than the motivation to exercise a separate subjectivity—anything to maintain the *status quo*. In a couple's middle years when two people could be freer of the stresses and strains of young children and uncertain careers, we often find that a false cordiality has substituted for intimate relating, hanging like a veil over difficult issues and muffling argument to the point where each member of the couple has turned elsewhere for gratification or becomes depressed. Where is the power here? Power in these situations can take the form of succumbing to the seductions of work and success, or residing in the making of fixed assumptions about ones partner's responses and thereby providing the powerful excuses for keeping secrets from the other. Secrets may then substitute for differentiation. Then, of course, there is the kind of communication between two people where one member of the couple renders the other utterly powerless in what I call a "relational (k)not" (Chapter 3). These knots, or negations, are so dense and untouchable that even the couple therapist may be rendered powerless.

Note this example: Stuart and I are sitting with an elderly couple. Part of their problem has to do with each of their disabilities. The husband, having suffered a stroke and using a walker, requires a good deal of care. His wife refuses outside help and tends to him resentfully and lovingly—enjoying the sense of being so needed. The trouble is, she is losing her hearing and also stubbornly refuses to purchase hearing aids. Although we understand the delicacy of this matter—it seems that spectacles are less threatening to a person's self and vanity than hearing aids—we feel that our effectiveness as therapists is somewhat compromised by having to shout our interventions. After one such effort on my part, the husband (H) repeated to his wife (W) what I had said, only louder:

W: I heard her. [*in a snapping tone*]
H: What did she say?
W: I told you, I heard!
H: You really should consider hearing aids.
W: I told you that I heard her. [*Her voice wavered. I imagined pain and humiliation. Glaring at her husband, she skirted whatever was going on inside her heart.*] You *insult* me with your continued insinuations about my hearing.

Helplessly, in an attempt at multilateral empathy, I intervened again. "We don't know whether he meant it as an insult, Mary," I shouted. "I'm almost totally blind. It really bothers me. I don't know what I'd do without my glasses."

"Well," she said, still glaring at her husband, "Some of us are blind, some of us are deaf, and some of us are *crippled*. I guess we just have to learn to live with what we're given."

The power here lies in the deniable negation. Mary says one thing and means another. On the surface she is a spokesperson for adaptation, but underneath the words she has returned her experience of her husband's insult in spades, and we feel like we have no way of touching it. Here, our silence is not the silence of containment or acceptance, it is the silence of a helpless retreat that is no doubt shared by Mary's husband.

Containment within a couple relationship is a very subtle business in the sense that, like a hunter's lair when shooting ducks, containment can double as a blind for avoidance, serve as a patronizing advantage in the light of another's open exposure, or both. Where acceptance is concerned, when two people are both simultaneously vulnerable and equally adamant, they are deaf to the idea of alternating care. The timed asymmetry required by such reciprocal exchange is out the window! How could it be otherwise?

If (given limited opportunity and space) I were permitted one generalization about how the intersubjective dialectic between power and intimacy goes slack in a way that cripples the transformative power of recognition, I would venture the notion that couples need to learn from the consulting room that you cannot fight and explore at the same time. Couples need to learn to distinguish fighting from exploring. Sometimes talking it out needs to wait awhile before the next session begins. When couples opt to fight, they need to learn how to fight fairly. There is a framework for this process—a set of general principles and boundaries (see the Appendix).

However, containment, acceptance, and recognition in a viable couple relationship also differ in experience and form from how we might describe their usefulness in the consulting room. For me, in my couple, this also means that I will *not* always be present. Sometimes, after a fight, I require my own sense of distance, space, and time, for which—in marriage—I am not charged, before I can return to my most prized relationship. In this sense, containment, acceptance, and recognition imply a kind of mutual trust in the ongoing future of true relating between us. I will be gone for an indeterminate while, and although I am at present not inclined in your direction, you and I can *trust* that I will be back. And I *must*, when I get back, without intending to cripple you with what you may at first reflexively perceive as wound, express what I feel or have felt directly—in a manner that I would never reveal to those with whom I have undertaken to explore in my role as therapist or analyst. Intimacy in the consulting room differs from intimacy in a couple. In the consulting room, two people are intimately and powerfully engaged in the exploration of one person's going on being. Engagement in a couple that continues to provide and maintain ongoing growth extends beyond the four walls of two people's asymmetrical efforts to be with and learn from one another. Actually, in that regard we find the expression, "we're trying to work harder and pay more attention to our relationship," as rather deadening in itself. Vitality in a couple comes through the discovery of new experiences in the outside world, new adventures undertaken separately or together—enriching a couple's life and conversation. Liveliness, of course, is not meant to take the place of clear communication in life partnerships or in therapeutic partnerships, where disclosures generally differ—in timing as well as degree of transparency.

Indirection, as I have already indicated, can also be an insidious form of taking power. My dad, an attorney, used to bitterly complain about how lawyers befuddle their clients, or remove themselves from what they are actually dealing with, by exercising the power of needlessly complex legalese. "Why," he used to say, "can't lawyers write in simple English?" He loved to parrot, as an example, the writing of a will. "Instead of all that 'hereby donate, bequeath, and so convey my personal effects,' why not just say, 'I leave my furniture to Joe.'"

For Stuart and myself, "I leave my furniture to Joe" has become a familial metaphor for valuing direct affective expressiveness between us. However, I would also add that a certain circularity, like flirting, adds music and color to ongoing relating. Stuart's use of humor and metaphor, for example, provides an intimate grace note in tough moments of personal despair or in the shadow of unrelenting tasks ahead. I remember one evening, when I was particularly looking forward to a night of quiet relaxation, Stuart came into my office at the end of the day with what struck me as a mile-long list of things we *had* to do that night. When he got to the last item, I leaned down on my desk to cup the burden of my head and, sighing between my open fingers, said, "And then I'll shoot myself!" To which Stuart, with a hand on my shoulder, softly replied, "I'd miss you, but … can I have your toys?" We both found relief in joint laughter.

That transformative moment notwithstanding, we were up and busy much later than we had hoped. As a consequence, Stuart, who had a bad cold already, slept fitfully that night. The combination of his snoring and my exhaustion kept me awake.

In conclusion, I illustrate just how I dealt with it—a testament, perhaps, to the transformative power of intimacy, a transformation that happens in those moments of balance in the dialectic between power and intimacy. I am talking about those inspiring moments both in the consulting room and in personal relationships when the heart of the matter comes closest to matters of the heart; when, as Susan Coates (1998) related, "a slight mismeeting allows a symbolic stance to occur and provides a creative spark" (p. 128).

That night of chores, the residue of joint laughter, Stuart's snoring, and my exhaustion led me to leave our bed and move upstairs. However, rather than sinking down into my cot, I found myself at the computer. This, would you believe, became what wrote itself in the dark of early morning:

SNORING

Most often will your
Snoring roar me
Like a distant ocean's
Stormy risings from the deep.
Your rhythmic wheezes
Come as such sweet lullabies
That I am sucked with you to sleep.

And yet this night my dear
You treat me to a
Veritable vaudeville show
Of scattered snorts complete
With bells and whistles,
Stuttered snaps and rattle taps
Along with breathless arcs
That spread through dark
Like imitation "scuttle" missiles.

And the minute I'm convinced
You'll even out, you start anew
Engaging me in sudden giggles
With your pig-sty sound bites
As you syncopate your sighs
With purse of lips that whoop
And oops and snort and pew …

Darling, you must know by now
How much I love you more and more
With every breath you take,
I promise that I'll try my best
To go to sleep but just in case,

If I should die before you wake
I hope you'll take my
Will without a blow.
So help me God, though I am yours—
I leave my toys to Joe!

Appendix
Fighting Fair

Here are a few examples of principles and boundaries:

- No turning the tables in the moment of your partner's complaint (e.g, "Well, you do it too").
- No bringing up of your partner's vulnerabilities for the sake of scoring a point (power play) in the moment.
- No upping the *ante* with a list of grievances from the past (another power play).
- No moving from substance to *ad hominem.*
- Try to repeat your understanding of your partner's grievance before responding to it.
- Try to stick to "I" statements.
- Try to avoid the "well you always" and "you never" rebuttals. Stay on target with the current issue.
- Try to recognize when your partner has made you too angry to fight fair and call a time out.

Couples may build in their own rules and regulations for fighting fair. And it *is* fair for one to remind the other when one of these rules is broken. It is also a signal for time out.

Notes

1 An earlier version of this article was presented at the sixteenth annual conference, "Behind Closed Doors: The Power of Intimacy in the Personal and Analytic Relationship," National Institute for the Psychotherapies, New York, February 5, 2005, and at a conference of the same title at the Institute of Contemporary Psychoanalysis, Los Angeles, September 17, 2005.
2 A version of this case material was previously published in B. Pizer (2000).
3 See also Mitchell's (2000) elaboration of this point in *Relationality: From Attachment to Intersubjectivity* (p. 133).

4 This version is an excerpt in altered form from my "Interpretive Activity, Destruction and Recognition: A Dialogue with Lawrence Brown," presented at the Boston Institute for Psychotherapy Symposium, November 4, 2000, and dedicated to the late Dr. Julius Silberger.

5 See his chapters 8 and 9.

References

Coates, S. (1998). Having a mind of ones own and holding the other in mind. *Psychoanalytic Dialogues, 8*, 87–114.

Hoffman, I. Z. (1998). *Ritual and spontaneity in the psychoanalytic process*. Hillsdale, NJ: The Analytic Press.

McLaughlin, J. T. (1991). Clinical and theoretical aspects of enactment in the psychoanalytic situation. *Journal of the American Psychoanalytic Association, 39*, 595–614.

Mitchell, S. A. (2000). *Relationality: From attachment to intersubjectivity*. Hillsdale, NJ: The Analytic Press.

Oates, J. C. (1993). *"Avarice" in "seven deadly sins."* New York: *The New York Times Book Review*.

Pizer, B. (2000). The therapist's routine consultations: A necessary window in the treatment frame. *Psychoanalytic Dialogues, 10*, 197–207.

Pizer, B. (2003). When the crunch is a (k)not: A crimp in relational dialogue. *Psychoanalytic Dialogues, 13*, 171–192.

Pizer, S. A. (1998). *Building bridges: The negotiation of paradox in psychoanalysis*. Hillsdale, NJ: The Analytic Press.

Reverie

I'll Never Forget

I'll never forget the night my dad didn't beat me. I remember how he came crashing into my room, grabbed the magazine out of my hand, threw it on the pile next to me, and stood me up at the same time. He may have been drinking, but I can't swear to it. Then he had both his big hands on each side of my shirt collar, pulling me up even closer to his face. "Well, son," he hissed, "what do you have to say for yourself?"

And I had to work real hard not to burst out laughing. For two reasons. The first is that my dad, as I may have said, is a big man, and I felt terrified over what he was going to do to me. And the second reason I wanted to laugh is because I found those magazines under his side of the bed, and I could have said the same thing to him.

DOI: 10.4324/9781032666303-14

A Clinical Exploration of Moving Anger Forward

Intimacy, Anger, and Creative Freedom

Part 1: Introduction: Anger and Potential

When it comes right down to it, I find it hard to write about the subject of anger, particularly as it pertains to the patient who had to leave treatment. She came in saying that she'd been much too angry all her life. She kept getting into trouble—anger spilling out all over people whom she barely knew. Something was the matter with her and she didn't know what. Always out of control. After about a month of seeing her I suggested that maybe she hadn't been angry enough to begin with. She asked me how I came to say what I said, and I didn't know how to tell her it was just my feeling. And I certainly didn't know her well enough to say the feeling was uncomfortably familiar.

So there it is. Being gripped by something that I can't quite grasp gives me the impetus to try to explain what I mean when I talk about the two-way track that anger may take, the inherent fallout from anger disavowed, and the potential vitality that emerges with ownership of anger, including the creative possibilities and risks involved in the process of moving anger forward toward more intimate relating.

My mother—who held her anger back along with many of the rest of her feelings—let me know that even though she loved me as much as her other daughters, I was definitely the problem child. She found me oversensitive and temperamental. Whenever I got angry or particularly upset, I felt her disappear. In calmer moments she would try to explain what made my "fits" so unbearable for her. Since she was born and raised in Europe with English as her second language, she couldn't make sense of my angry messages or find the words to soothe my pain. Naturally, I took in her trouble as failures of my own while at the same time feeling unable to help myself. More than anything, I yearned for her closeness. But the overall message I received

DOI: 10.4324/9781032666303-15

was that I "could never get enough, was never satisfied." It seemed to me no matter how hard I tried to please, I would forever be a stranger in my family. I felt bad. And also mad.

Maybe this "person or people hunger" combined with shame-faced loneliness contributed to the care and feeding of my avid interest in psychoanalytic studies. Imagine my relief on reading Winnicott's (1971) formulations of aggression as intrinsic to maturational processes! The "good-enough" mother's nonretaliatory survival of her baby's destructive moves allows him to place her outside of his omnipotent control, creating the rich potential of a *shared* reality between two separate subjectivities. Henceforth, the limitations of intrapsychic processes, the internal workings of connection or disconnection are awarded the broader possibilities offered by intersubjective experience.

Referring to the clinical setting, Epstein (1984) elaborated the analytic task in the face of overt or covert aggression by making substantial use of Winnicott's (1990/1971) ideas,[1] which he quotes:

> "Without the experience of maximum destructiveness (object not protected) the subject never places the analyst outside (of the area of omnipotent control) and therefore can never do more than experience a kind of self-analysis using the analyst as a projection part of the self. In terms of feeding, the patient then, can feed only on the self and cannot use the breast for getting fat. The patient may even enjoy the analytic experience but will not fundamentally change." (Winicott quoted in Epistein, p. 652)

With gratitude to Winnicott, Epstein, and those clinician/theorists who have already charted significant aspects of my terrain (and I mean to quote from a few of them as I go along), this chapter, including a clinical illustration, explores both linking and unlinking potentials carried by anger.

In our work with patients' repetitive patterns fueled by anger, we note the unlinking of affect from cognition in an unconscious operation that we call dissociation in one form or another, or dissociative patterns that we have come to recognize as the repetition compulsion. Inevitably, something angry making in the treatment situation, something too terrible to take occurs, causing a reflexive cut in connection. We assume that some past experience has been conflated and ironed down like a stencil in the mind through which our patient's present and future appear unalterably viewed. I agree with Russell's (2006a) notion that, "functionally, we can understand the repetition compulsion as a resistance to affect, to remembering with feeling" (p. 87). But that is not the whole of it exactly. *We tend to overlook the role of anger as it relates to cognition in the unlinking process*, which Russell rightly and precisely subsumes along with other component dimensions of affect.

Only recently have I learned more about the role of cognitive unlinking in an article from the Center for Research on Bilingualism in the United Kingdom, and published in the *Journal of Neuroscience* (Wu & Thierry, 2012, pp. 6485–6489). Apparently experimental psychology already has clarified that the bilingual human mind—when reading second-language words—spontaneously activates native language translation. It is also known that "emotional content is a fundamental part of language based communication" (p. 6485). But this current study offers surprising evidence of what happens when Chinese bilingual subjects are presented English words like *war*, *violence*, and other related angry words conveying *a negative valence*. Researchers Wu and Thierry have succeeded in unraveling emotional arousal from linguistic access through a complex experimental design involving careful collection of behavioral and electrophysiological data. Results show that emotions conveyed by potentially disturbing words "trigger *inhibitory mechanisms* that *block access* to the native language" (p. 6485, emphasis added). Thus we might infer that my mother's assessment of her difficulty had been on target after all. And of course there is more to it, which may account for the boldface title of Wu and Thierry's article proclaiming, "**How Reading in a Second Language Protects Your Heart**."

There is more to say about this research, but for the moment let's simply hold on to the hypothesis that higher order intellectual processes are innately intertwined with the language of the heart; that the components of emotion, including perception, intention, memory, and a variety of affect's cognitive functions (see Russell, 2006b), are all a part of the affective inborn interweave of mind/body/brain, a unity or balance that seems impossible to maintain. Much of what we do in our consulting rooms is to try to understand what causes the person we are sitting with to feel "unhinged," or unhinge us. In hindsight we attempt to mark the moment when dissociation takes us over (see Russell, 2006b; see also Bromberg, 2006, 2012; D. B. Stern, 1997, 2010), or when our patient disconnects.

From the beginning of my work in this field, my analytic sensibility has been rooted in the assumption of an innate impetus within each one of us to discover or restore our own unique balance of affective cognitions, and the thrust of my analytic inquiry is based on the inevitable breakdowns in cognitive-affective linking, breakdowns that hamper our thoughts about what we are feeling and interfere with the feel of whatever it is we may be thinking.

I am reminded of myself as a young child, sitting by my mother enjoying a warm sense of pleasure as I watched her nursing my baby sister. It was as if her more usually opaque countenance had magically transformed and I thought of her as "coming into her face." Then came the day that she was suddenly locked away behind her bedroom door. I remember a bustling in the hall where I hung around waiting. After a while my stomach began to ache as I tried not to hear the strange uneven sounds of raspy breath—was she choking? Or could it be that my inexpressive mother was sobbing in there? No way for me to reach her. The doctor came and the doctor went, gently closing the door behind him. Our family doctor. The familiar lingering scent on him, of his hands as he drummed the knuckles of two fingers against the flat of his hand on my chest, then tapped around my neck as if it were a keyboard, had always been such a comfort but now that antiseptic smell was uncontained— permeating our hallway, invading through the crack of my mother's bedroom door like I was standing in the sickening corridor of a hospital.

I don't remember when my mother finally came out of her room, but I noticed that she never nursed again. Or talked to me about what happened. I do remember in that unspoken time I vowed to really try and hold my anger in, do a better job with my tantrums.

There are no sensible words to describe the total experience of what I am trying to convey— only a visceral memory connected to the heave and rasp of mother's breath, the hospital smell, and a strong sense that my interest in breakdowns may have originated here.

We realize that affective-cognitive unlinking may save us in situations of early relational trauma or any trauma for that matter. We literally incapacitate ourselves for the sake of survival. But how might "survival" evolve toward reintegration and growth?

I am particularly intrigued by the ways in which the affect of anger— so often driven by fear or terror—may serve both unlinking and relinking functions. An unexpected upsurge of anger carries the potential to move us forward in an integrative way toward personal freedom and subsequent intimacy or may just as easily undo us, breaking off connections within ourselves as well as with others. For purposes of this exploration, let's conceive of cognitive-affective dissociation (elsewhere I have referred to it as cognitive flummoxing)[2] or repetition compulsion as a second-order code signifying unlinked primary occurrences that we have been unable either to get our heads around or to feel (see also B. Pizer, 2003). Repeated over and over, this personal verbal or nonverbal code becomes a familiar second language that we speak, hear, and enact, implicitly or explicitly, until otherwise notified by some surprise or new experience.

For some reason, we tend to think of repetition as it plays out in our enactments, but I believe the more subtle repetition is related to the way we *hear* the messages that come to us and how we formulate our reply.

We will notice later, in the unfolding of my case illustration, one example of the consequences that ensue when a patient's or analyst's affective intentions or wants are colored and ultimately marooned inside the procedural grammar of her second language. This second language or repetitive cognitive code is unlinked from patient's or analyst's primary connectedness with perception, intention, feeling, thinking, communicating, remembering, and so on.

As I said, I am currently focused on the power of anger and its role in facilitating or breaking down connections between affect and cognition. At just about the time I became more actively engaged in exploring the phenomenon, I received an invitation to speak at a conference. Along with this event, I was approaching the end of my work with a woman from another country whom I greatly admired and who had entered therapy for the brief duration of her Visitor's Permit in the United States. It is important for an understanding of what follows to note that although my patient was born and grew up in another country, her parents were British and she was raised with English as her primary mode of communication. I realized that she brought us a long-term project—beginning with the business of recognizing the origins of unharnessed aggression, but I could not resist the opportunity to work with her. And as the time grew closer to our arbitrary termination, I grew sadder that we could not move further with the task I thought we had so well begun.

Then, in the process of choosing a clinical vignette to illustrate the ideas I had set down, it suddenly occurred to me that maybe if I wrote about our mutual effort, we could continue somehow by correspondence. I would send her drafts of what I wrote and she would send her comments back. The notion of continuing collaboration clearly pleased her, pleased us both.

"Yes," she said, she really liked the idea. Nevertheless, we thought it wise to take more time to think about it. Over a weekend before she left I sent her a tentative trial draft that described an impasse and our brief but incomplete foray into an angry exchange.

Quite rightly, my patient complained that I had not sufficiently disguised her, but as for the dialogue, her only comment was "What happens next?"

Once I addressed those issues in an immediate e-mail reply, I wrote, "I fear that foreshortened time has prompted in me a premature push for enactment. I would like to write about us (and yes, with you as disguised as you might want and deserve to be) as a way of preserving some aspect of an experience that I hold precious, but more than that. Something for you too. And larger than the both of us maybe. Maybe a contribution to this field of work."

Looking at it now, I think to myself, "How grandiose!" I continue.

"BUT please know that I don't want to 'use you.' Or exploit our work because our work is more important to me, and I hope to you. And if 'exploitation' or 'misuse' comes into your mind, please let me know."

In our next session, still a few weeks before our final goodbye, my patient denied suspicion over being exploited. She regarded our experiment as a gift and wanted to continue.

But what could either of us have really known?

Only much later would I come to understand that my failures in this treatment—among them, denial of anger over our separation paired with a decided inability to recognize the disconnect it prompted—buckled us both.[3]

And so we continued our project long distance. I just cannot imagine my foolhardiness! I cannot get away from the truth of my enacted breakdown between emotional and thinking processes. I should have thought better than to engage my patient in a collaborative venture to outline unfinished business as a way of naming whatever anger we could find between us, as an example of a mutual effort to move shared anger forward. How absurd! Indeed, we kept in intermittent contact as I sent her drafts.

As I awaited response to my final draft, I finally felt the apprehension that something had gone wrong between my former patient and me. Her angry e-mail came on the eve of my departure, and I left for the conference armed with a presentation that, in the very last minute, I could not possibly deliver.

Including my introduction, I have divided this chapter into three parts. Part 2 is an excerpted version of the presentation I gave as substitute for the one I trashed on arrival in the conference city.

In Part 3, I clarify my former patient's responses to the revised presentation. I present my view of how the acknowledgment of anger between us led to an unexpected outcome. I talk about what I believe to be the meaning of moving anger forward. In so doing, I also draw inferences from that research reported in the *Journal of Neuroscience* (2012) suggesting the presence of a cognitive marker for screening negative affective words. As summarized in the Medicalxpress (Bangor University, 2012),

> This finding breaks new ground in our understanding of the interaction between emotion and thought in the brain. Previous work on emotion and cognition has already shown that emotion affects basic brain functions such as attention, memory, vision and motor control, but never at such a high processing level as language and understanding.

Finally, I leave it to you whether or not you agree with my belief that despite the limited time we had together, and even if I never see my former patient again, there is evidence that some transformation actually has taken place between us.

Part 2: The Therapist's Use of Self

I am about to give you a living example of moving anger forward. My own. On the day before I left town fully prepared to deliver a paper, or so I thought, I received an e-mail from another country where my former patient is a citizen. Originally she had wholeheartedly agreed to my presenting our project. But in the last minute, she changed her mind.

It has been six months now since she had to leave treatment. The treatment ended prematurely, but we both knew in advance that she would be called back home. Although in a previous e-mail she expressed her gratitude—citing a recent achievement as example of her progress (unfortunately, taking no credit for her part), telling me, "I always liked talking with you.... I would not have lasted through [my stay in the US] without that support." Receipt of my final draft completely turned the tables. What a shock.

So here I am, still reeling and, in an effort to move my own anger forward, still wanting to explore with you the role of anger in intersubjective relating, particularly when genuine intimacy—or my illusion of that shared self-state—unfolds between analyst and patient.

Even though I am unable to flesh out the person I planned to talk about, I believe all the more that our experience together—which she in this moment repudiates—emphasizes the significance, variation, and influence of anger in human relationships, highlighted by analytic interchange.

As I become clear enough to reflect on my former patient's change of heart around my former paper, I see that, in a way, her withdrawal is not really a legitimate part of analytic interchange. At best, I have to take responsibility for having created the enactment without a context to contain it. Looking back I can see that my own personal grief over the arbitrary loss of our connection had a lot to do with the wish to set down something of my view of what transpired between us. A way of holding.

The central issue around which I believed our work revolved and around which this chapter still revolves has to do with anger, intimacy, and the release of creative freedom as these factors apply to analytic work. I believe that genuine intimacy between patient and analyst is dependent on the ability of both partners to trust their ongoing process, with trust being contingent on the degree to which each participant can recognize, metabolize, and ultimately express angry emotions directly to one another.

Much has been made of the curative power of *analytic love*. For me, there is too much bestowal in it, too much potency given over to the analyst. For me, the therapeutic work and play lie in finding common pathways that lead toward an acceptable degree of intimacy between participants. Analytic intimacy begins with the analyst's ability to be herself as analyst, to discover moment by moment who that self is in relation to each patient and to be with what each patient brings to the interaction (see Russell, 1996). As I define it, this kind of intimacy between analyst and patient takes its own sweet time, is neither preordained nor static but rather a genuinely felt ongoing back and forth, a moment-by-moment negotiation of closeness and distance. Intimate analytic relating in this asymmetrical context involves the gradual achievement of mutual engagement, including the ability to recognize and metabolize angry emotions. Above all else, the process takes time.

Back to *analytic love*: There's that one aspect of the concept that sets my teeth on edge. Of course it's true that analytic love *happens* between ourselves and our patients as intimacy along with trust is developed in the consulting room, and we talk about it in terms of defining the boundaries and the setting in which these often-necessary or unavoidable or joyous affects do occur. Stephen Mitchell's (2000)[4] groundbreaking essay about love and hate in the clinical context is an important asset in our theoretical and technical literature. Nevertheless there's a danger embedded in the concept also that we can't ignore, a tinge of power there, a one-up/one-down tendency that we have to be careful of (see Chapter 9).

So even though it might be true that "love makes the world go round," there is also the reality that unconscious and untended aggression in the name of love or cure or saving the world threatens to blow our world apart. Whatever political action we might take in the service of peace in the world, whatever else each of us may try to do to stop the spread of violence perpetrated by power for power's sake, the quieter more organizing process[5] of human growth and *being* is, I believe, indispensable, and that requires self-awareness—including an awareness of the roots of our aggression in the context of intimate relating.

My ire rises as I think now about my former patient who seems to consider the paper I wrote as an insult—the paper I thought was a document in which my warmth, my foibles, and empathic caring came through as did our mutual efforts to make sense of her dilemma. My former patient is furious, but the fury is ice cold, the kind that frightens me, the kind that leaves me feeling three years old and wanting to appease. But she views the work as a one-up/one-down exposé in which I paint her as "hapless" and me as a "success"! How could she?

But then again, why is it that we analysts so often forget about transference dynamics— *working both ways I hasten to add*—when we feel we are being so authentic (how I hate that word)! Or maybe the way in which we think we are being real is actually thoughtless, hurtful, judgmental, bullying, inattentive.

I am finding in this anger that I'm trying to move forward confusion as to who is who and who is doing what to whom? "Did I do this or was it done to me?" (See Russell, 1975/2006d, p. 14; 1987/2006a, p. 46.)

I can remember like yesterday that freezing winter afternoon when fifth grade let out, and the class bully, Alice Belerian, suddenly grabbed hold of me from behind and pushed me down on my knees and rubbed my face in the snow. I can remember running home crying, to tell my mother, sobbing that Alice Belerian pushed me in the snow—to which my mother coolly replied, "And what did you do to her?"

For me the track of my emotional reactions usually moves from hurt and anger to shame and hurt, and then in rapid fire, to the rescue, I design an angry fantasy that gets me back up on my feet again.

Hopefully for analyst or therapist, the process of acknowledging her anger—while aware of her powerful role in the dyad—takes the form of an internal negotiation (see also S. Pizer, 1992) or conversation. I believe that the patient will pick up the analyst's implicit struggles and make of them what she can bear at the time. And hopefully, in her good time, the patient will begin to feel safe enough to express what she feels directly to the analyst, including her feelings of anger. And here I risk the statement that genuine trust cannot be fully attained without identifying, engaging, working through, and surviving direct expressions fueled by anger. Simple anger, according to Guntrip's (1971) definition, is a defense against assault (p. 37). As first response, anger serves an adaptive function. A responsive upsurge of anger may become a clarifying signal in relationship, a statement of personal boundary that defines for the other the degree of closeness or distance permitted in this particular moment.

Somewhere inside, both parties in the analytic enterprise will know that trust between them remains incomplete and contingent until they have each expressed and received exchanges directly and consciously fueled by anger and together lived through its shared experience.

As Mitchell (1998) wrote, "So we can begin with the hypothesis that each patient (and each analyst as well) is likely to experience, either consciously or unconsciously, one or more versions of themselves as quite destructive, sadistic, and vengeful" (p. 28). And so,

> One important task of analysis is to create an atmosphere in which that version of self can come to life, become known, so that the patient can become better able to contain and to be reconciled with the various versions of self, including destructive versions. From this perspective, therefore, one cannot simply work on or through aggression indirectly because in so doing, one bypasses a full immersion in and conscious processing of important domains of self experience. (pp. 28–29, emphasis added)

Is it not ironic, then, that my former patient's responses to me that came out of a draft I sent her (purported understanding that morphed in cyberspace into misunderstanding both ways) led to expressions of anger between us that neither of us could fully feel in vivo? We missed the freedom that we both had wished for, the creative freedom between us that just might have been. If only we had had the time!

Makes me mad. "I'm rubber, you're glue," I am thinking to tell my former patient now, "Whatever you say jumps off of me and sticks to you." Okay, so I'm behaving like a baby now. "Well, you can go jump in a lake!!"

Almost immediately, I turn myself around. "This is hubris. All your fault." I am hugely ashamed. Now to the whole world at large, "You know what she said," I parrot on, "she said, 'You didn't listen … you seem to have been thinking about yourself all the time." And I turn around again. *"But I'm all I have left, dumbbell, now that you took yourself away, you can just go jump in a lake!"*

I know that when my feelings move in that direction, I am sunk if I let them go down. The internal landscape is barren and familiar. At bottom I feel caught out, ashamed beyond belief, maybe for having set the whole thing up in the first place, so all I can do is blather diatribes inside my head to muster up the energy that anger provides. Some energy to pull myself together.

Clearly anger comes in various flavors and may help or hinder whatever it is we wish for in our lives; anger may be growth producing, creative, protective, defensive, or destructive. Although we know that all of us are born with the capacity to feel, *owning* whatever the feeling is that wells up inside is something else entirely. Recognition, acceptance, and creative use of one's anger may be one of our most difficult developmental tasks.

And now, I continue to think about my former patient, about how proud I felt when I sent her that last draft, an ongoing sense of pride until she set me straight. And I can feel in my body the way her response turned pride into an in-breath of shocked surprise, then a metabolic drop into the place of hurt with, I realize in retrospect, a brief pit stop in the area of outrage. I'd get back to anger later on.

I want to say that by pride I don't mean the hubris kind that "goeth before the fall," but rather a very personal and private sense of empowerment, a kind of anchoring integrity that comes from behaving in concert with one's felt beliefs, a pride that actually may manifest itself as a rising warmth inside. Feeling proud can be an emotion like anger, too often bred out of us "lest it go to our heads" or give reason to lose one's temper, heaven forbid. And again I am reminded of my mother's comment when Alice Belerian took me down. Perhaps the consequence of receiving automatic and unjust blame is that it feeds the idea that anger must be justified before one has a right to feel it. And then what follows may be the insidious merger of anger with judgment that sends a person so far away from spontaneity and trust that should you happen to ask her what she's feeling, she will shrug and tell you, "Nothing." And soon she will believe it, experiencing nothing at all or something else. It could well be that some degree of trust must be established before patient (or therapist) dares to test her anger in an analytic setting. Most likely it works both ways. Just as the affects of love and hate bear a close relationship with one another, so too may anger and trust.

You know, just as I am beginning to think you must be getting bored with all this exploration, this focus on inner process that right now relates only to me, but I hope has relevance to you as well, I see that even though I hold myself responsible for having caused my former patient anguish, I am separating, slowly, from her global assessment.

I do remember sitting with her on a winter day, and we were talking deeply about a history of growing up that left her with the kind of scars that maybe one could overcome to some degree, make some creative use of their enduring ache (and isn't that what we as therapists routinely do, what makes us therapists in the first place?) but scars that just won't ever go away. I can feel the way it was as we sat together enveloped in a long silence. I was filled with a mixture of experience for which I had no words, perhaps because my own reveries had fallen away. The way I felt with her was a way I had not felt before—a depth of pain that could just as easily have flopped over into joy, a very quiet and connected place where—as in dreams—opposite feelings intertwine, a timeless place. Outside my window it had just begun to snow—thick random flakes.

Even if today she will deny it ever happened, even if the thing is only a figment of my imagination, even if I need it as a source of solace, I can feel it inside, and it belongs to me—next to my anger and my sadness and whatever else there is.[6]

And now I have arrived at yet a new place. I recognize that anger is more than just a feeling. Anger may also be a mode of transportation that carries with it a richness of unexpected feelings as it travels along, feelings and combinations of feelings never felt in quite this way before or again. And stepping back, I also realize that anger, like laughter, moves us out of dissociation and into the present moment.

My former patient puts me in a lineup with the other figures who betrayed her, and that makes me feel *shut out*. According to Guntrip (1971), "Aggression can be a meaningful reaction to bad object relations," and if the paper triggered my patient into a state that Guntrip talks about when he speaks of "aggression that changes into frustrated rage, hate, fear, and flight" (p. 37), then maybe I need to take it personally in the sense that I may not be its object, but I do, in a way, need to stand alongside of her lineup of perpetrators. I feel sad and responsible for that.

I think of Liotti's (2004) summary of Blizard's 2001 research that high-lights the paradoxical relational dilemma following attachment disorgan-ization. "In order to maintain attachment, traumatic memories of abuses suffered at the hands of family members must be dissociated, but to protect the self from abuse, the need for attachment must be disavowed" (p. 483). How then could my former patient ever really feel the fullness of her anger with me directly? How could she ever trust relationship? Yes, we needed more time.

Before I close, I want to quote from Guntrip (1971) as a way of empha-sizing the importance of working analytically with anger for the sake of greater creative freedom and the development of intimacy.

In summary, Guntrip (1971) argued against Freud's notion that aggres-sion and destructiveness constitute a primary instinctive drive. *He pointed out that "the more primitive the society, the more aggression becomes sim-ply self-defense"* (p. 120, emphasis added).

And yet even today we hang on to the idea of training our children to disown anger and natural aggression. Many of us grow up with the idea that anger directly expressed is primitive. We need to relearn anger as integral to being real, a necessary ingredient of intimate relating.

Guntrip (1971) wrote,

The more complex societies become, the more fears and insecurities cre-ate vicious circles of suspicion, defensiveness, defenses by attack and counterattack. An aggressive society becomes self-perpetuating, a nearly insoluble problem. But we must not blindly ascribe this to nature and instinct.

It is a sign of the bankruptcy of the creative capacities to live and love. Being, the sense of assured stable selfhood, is the basis of healthy doing, of spontaneous creative activity. Without it, doing can only be forced self-driving to keep oneself going, a state of mind that breeds aggres-sion, in the first place against oneself, and then to gain some relief from self-persecution, it is turned outward against other people, situations, or causes, creating the social neuroses of fanaticism, political, religious, or idiosyncratic. (p. 120)

As I go over my notes about the work with my former patient, I still believe that we touched her anger and her pain together, or at least I did. I *know I did*. But we didn't have the time to hold it long enough in the room between us for her to metabolize it in the present. Whether my former patient will ever forgive me or ever completely "get" what I'm trying to articulate is an open question. I have no idea what or how much she will ultimately hang on to from the time we spent. As for my experience, I can say without a doubt that a dimension of feeling has opened in me that had not been there before, a feeling as real and as evanescent as the first fall of snow outside my office window.

Part 3: Time to Hold It Long Enough?

As for other, more familiar dimensions of feeling, Mitchell (1998) unreservedly declared, "All of us experienced enough danger and threat in childhood, regardless of the balance of health or pathology in our caretakers, to have experienced at least a fair amount of destructive aggression. It is universal to hate," he insists, to "contemplate revenge against, and want to destroy those very caretakers we also love." Accordingly, in Mitchell's view, "one would start with the hypothesis that each patient (and each analyst as well) is likely to experience, either consciously or unconsciously, one or more versions of themselves as quite destructive, sadistic, and vengeful" (p. 28).

Given this universal yet "out-of-line" self-organization that wants to hide without a passport and no place to go, Mitchell prescribed an analytic antidote, which is worth repeating. He wrote

> One important task of analysis is to create an atmosphere in which that version of self can come to life, become known, so that the patient can become better able to contain and to be reconciled with the various versions of self, including destructive versions. From this perspective, therefore, one cannot simply work on or through aggression indirectly because, in so doing, one bypasses a full immersion in and conscious processing of important domains of self experience. (pp. 28–29, emphasis added)

I knew I would show my former patient how her anger with me worked for me. Our angry exchange did not destroy either of us, but her anger carried enough potency to influence and bring about change. The new version of my paper honored her objections, and I sent it off to her right away.

In contrast to the preceding fiasco, my former patient replied almost immediately. The powerful directness she now invested in her e-mail arguments struck me as a familiar part of who she is and was, but when she sat with me in person, I felt it only as a shadow. All I had to go on was a procedural sense of empathy and strength of purpose that crossed her face, so quickly followed by despair. I mean I felt her integrity even though the conflicts she now expressed in writing led to certain conclusions I could not endorse. It was the integrity of my former patient's character that I believed in, that drew me to engage with her in the first place, that didn't want to let her go before we could glue that portion of her being onto the wobbly places of self-doubt.

But that last-minute wish of mine (yes, my repetition) is just where I went wrong. Bromberg (2012) talked about "conditions for healing" (p. 274) in order for growth to occur, and those conditions have to do with "the ability to flexibly tolerate the presence of separate self-states simultaneously" (p. 274). It's a process that takes time and trust, and I had wishfully hoped we could defy our arbitrary termination by continuing in cyberspace.

As it happens, sending my former patient this new version of my paper surprisingly released the emergence of separate self-states all together. In reading my former patient's e-mail, I get a glimpse of gratitude, disdain, appreciation, reproach, global self-criticism, discrete awareness of self and other, and awareness of progress from then to now. But there is no one "standing in the spaces" (Bromberg, 1998) with her when she relays to me these separate self-states making simultaneous appearances in the same three e-mail pages like orphans taking issue in a play of words.

My former patient writes directly about her anger with me. "This time," she writes, "I thought about it hard and tried to say clearly what I was angry about." And, "I thought this change in my behavior was a sign of progress."

Then another self talks back, unlinking from the first. My former patient tells me how closely what happened with us mirrors those ruptured relationships with important people in her past who judged her every time she opened up, whose scathing diatribes and righteously demolishing "verdicts" denied all ownership of their negativity. As I read the gathering in of this self's condensed version of formative figures, their mystifying denials of anger while skewering her with "constructive criticism," I become aware of the key to the breakdown point in my former patient's development of cognitive-affective links.

I believe that my former patient's silenced self, which I have come to regard as closest to her core self, absorbed the aggregate of all demolishing "verdicts," holding them in procedural knowledge. And because of their deniability, she could never address them; never learn to address them directly. Now, in the transference, I wear the mantel of assassinator. Here is the precise point of disconnection, or relational trauma, which Russell (2006e) defined "in terms of the interruption of a containing relationship in the service of the capacity to feel" (p. 614). So my former patient can apprehend but she cannot yet link, because she dreads reprisals if she finds the language to speak what she feels.

But like any person hostage to the repetition compulsion, she knows what she "wants": to smoke out the disowned, demolishing intention in the response of the other. She must sustain such vigilance to survive in life, and in the transference. And yet, my former patient also has moved beyond the point from which she also continues to react. Her e-mail message speaks from multiple self-states that are unlinked, partially or tenuously linked, at the threshold of linkage. She writes, "This is clearly an old repetition, there's no getting around it." She writes, "I have learned not to express anger because the results are like this: not give and take but total repudiation." Here the silenced self gives me clues to her defensive retreat.

My former patient communicates with me from within our transference-countertransference repetitions and also from a perch of reflectiveness beyond it. She is capable of important, yet still intermittent, translation. But the lingering repetition continues to speak—unlinked, linked, unlinked.

In the throes of the repetition compulsion, a person *knows* what she wants but cannot see its disconnection from what she needs. My former patient *knew* she entered therapy wanting my verdict. In her e-mail, she writes, "I wanted to know what was wrong with me.... You tried, I think, to do what I wanted. But you never gave me the verdict, or even any friendly advice. The problem I came in with, I took away." I agree that, concretely, this is the case. But would my verdict move her anger forward? I believe that what she wanted was for me to collude with her so that she could remain safely silent in my compliance with her repetition. But I was guided by my belief that she needed a potential space for her own voice —to address *directly* her own anger in a recognizing relationship. Before receiving my revised paper, and in it my open anger, she struggled to regulate safety and change by expressing her need to stop my work on the paper. And, in the last minute, she found the courage to do it! Our separate enactments—my wish to continue our work by writing about it through exchanges with her and her silent tactic of delaying to stop me—surfaced our impasse. And by this courageously direct aggressive action, she broke through her silence and approached the realization that she could word, voice, and deliver unmitigated anger toward me. Although my explicit anger, as she found it in my paper, furthers the integrative process, this is essentially in the service of solidifying the important and freeing step that she herself had to take: to find and state her own anger directly in her first language.

Seeing this in writing underlines a felt sense of my own blind transference urgency to speed the process, the clumsy reach of my repetition through the door of her repetition that she could not yet open in order to link up to her own capacity for "self-other wholeness" (Bromberg, 2012, p. 276). As Bromberg wrote, "Self-other wholeness will be compromised early in life by developmental trauma that has no cognitive representation because *developmental trauma is attachment-related and organized procedurally rather than symbolically*" (p. 276).

Here I want to describe how cognitive researchers Wu and Thierry (2012) defined a perspective on this procedural organization in terms of the brain's capacity to inhibit language access. In their 2012 study of bilinguals, they have investigated the effect of affective valence on language access rather than the effect of affective processing per se. They presented Chinese bilinguals with a series of positive- and negative-affective English words that registered no difference of arousal in their subjects. However, subjects did not spontaneously translate the negatively valenced words, suggesting "emotional processing interacts in a *preventive* manner, automatically repressing full realization of semantic integration when the targeted meaning is potentially distressing" (p. 6489). Wu and Thierry thus concluded that their present findings "break new ground as regards emotion-cognition interactions" (p. 6489).

If we can agree to the metaphor of the repetition compulsion as a secondary code, can we infer that my patient's contradictory understandings around anger are also related to her difficulty in actually accessing love and hate in her primary or procedural connections to a language of love? Researcher Wu and Thierry (2012) contended,

> So far, insights into the spontaneous role of emotion on human cognition have been limited to basic cognitive processes such as attention,

memory, vision, and motor control. *Here we establish that emotional processing unconsciously interacts with cognitive mechanisms underlying language comprehension.* (p. 6489, emphasis added)

In writing, a part of my former patient is able to link up with what she perceived in my new version of the paper I presented. This part of her offers that she was impressed by my forthright approach to my colleagues, claiming that she wouldn't have had the courage. She says that she gained a greater understanding of how I saw the work with her in a way that she never did by reading our session notes (given to her on departure) or by reading the various versions of the paper I trashed.

She says she still doesn't know what I mean by "moving anger forward," even though it seems to be the central concept that I'm trying to get across.

The main lesson for her in our work, expressed by that part of her that must keep safe from change, is a lesson she learned from long ago, which is, *not* to express her anger in the presence of another person, particularly a woman. My angry revelations in the paper testify to what happens when you do.

I pause in this narrative to remind us of my brief introductory thoughts about the repetition compulsion—a cognitive-affective unlinking, a resistance to remembering with feeling (Russell, 2006c). More specifically, I elaborated a conception of the repetition compulsion as an enacted *code* for unlinked indigestible occurrences. I stated my belief that this personal code becomes a metaphor, a second language that gains increasing familiarity.

For Russell (1996), the repetition compulsion is "a psychological black hole from which the subject can see or feel no way out" (p. 212).

The patient was unable to experience then, and is unable to remember now, the traumatic event in the way that he needs to in order to be able to locate the event in the past, and be able to feel enough differently that the present and past can be distinguished. (p. 212)

My erstwhile patient oscillates between safety and risk. She tells me in her e-mail that she came to see me because she was tired of having to do everything herself, without support. So she was happy to come and talk to me. She acknowledges my efforts to do what she wanted. "You certainly tried …You did the work of two … took it off my shoulders." But still, she wanted to know what was wrong with her, and I "never gave [her] a verdict."

This self must insist that there is "something wrong" with her; she believes I have wholeheartedly expressed agreement with her detractors. When I speak of my fear of her cold fury, she hears me labeling her as a cold *person* altogether and thus incapable of expressing any other kind of anger; and when I spit back—in a hot, regressed, tantrumous, three-year-old rage—that she should "go jump in a lake," she feeds back to me that I wish her to drown; and when I quote Guntrip proposing the generalization that unprocessed anger handicaps human freedoms, she actually hears me to be proclaiming *along with Guntrip* that she is "incapable of life and love."

Holding Russell, Bromberg, and Wu and Thierry in mind, I read in my former patient's e-mail the degree of risk she actually took in presenting her anger to me. I experience in her concrete presentation of self-states how much therapeutic work she has actually done in the short time we had together as well as how much there is yet left to do. Our repetitions have been rendered in the cyberspace between us and, as life would have it, we are unable to see them through in the same space together. For the person I grew with for a short while, I believe that arrival at a reliable linking of past and present, memory and experience, want and need, affect and cognition remains an emergent potential. For now, she does know quite a lot about her relational and affective realities, but this knowledge remains primarily procedural, kept mostly private and safe behind closed doors—so far, untranslated. Moving anger forward takes continuing risk, disappointment, and surprise.

Moving anger forward, paradoxically, means also moving it back past coded repetitions where one may find in memory enough to go on to risk again communication of whatever has been already apprehended, and to speak up—in anger if needed—for oneself and one's boundaries with a trusted other.

Via e-mail, my former patient conveys in her anger with me that protective mechanisms of unlinking are still needed while at the same time she lets me in on her simultaneous linking. Her e-mail gives indication that some transformations, if ever so inchoate, have occurred between us.

Although she explicitly attributes inspiration to sources other than myself, she does let me know that she has allowed herself an inkling of surprise: "I came to you in the first place because I could not work. And you kept telling me I'd start soon as a result of our work. That didn't happen. But after I expressed my anger about your paper, something changed. I just realized I was on my own, as always, and I better get on with it." And then, she lets me know that even before receiving my revision, "I intended to e-mail and tell you that I started working again."

Acknowledgments

Special thanks to Hazel Ipp for her influence, steadfast support, and fine editing of this chapter. Thanks also to Donnel B. Stern for his encouragement and helpful comments on an earlier version. And I thank Stuart Pizer for his invaluable contribution to my work and the development of this chapter.

Notes

1 See *Playing and Reality*, Chapter 6, "The Use of an Object and Relating through Identifications" (p. 91).
2 See B. Pizer (2000).
3 Although one could say that in growing up, the parenting I received was far less toxic than my patient's, in the transference-countertransference matrix, we share a particular denial of anger with its accompanying move towards compliance that Epstein (1984, 1999) names as the employment of "implosive defences." Epstein (1999) wrote, "In most cases the patient was very early recruited by one or both parents to meet the parent's need. The sensitivity of these patients to the needs, feelings, and desires and vulnerability of others is such that it eclipses awareness of their own needs, feelings and desires. I think of them as being imprisoned in their empathy for others. They tend to be hypocritical of themselves, self-hateful" (p. 311).
4 Mitchell's (2000) paper bears the title "Intersubjectivity: Between Expressiveness and Restraint in the Analytic Relationship." In this context, it is important not to ride over Mitchell's dialectical truth that "expressiveness" includes hate as well as love. Furthermore, in an earlier paper, Mitchell (1998) asserted that aggression arises "not as a bolster of a singular, essentially non-aggressive self, but as a central organizing component of one among multiple self-organizations" (p. 28).
5 See also Paul Russell (1976/2006a) on owning affects and negotiating affects. These become the developmental structures inherent to the growth of human being and constitute "a quieter, more powerful" organizing process" (p. 626).
6 Although delivered too late (and not in person), my efforts to understand and own my contribution to our transference/countertransference impasse inadvertently opened a space that had an impact that I would not realize until sometime later. Epstein (1999) tells us, "Whether the analyst's emotional vulnerability turns out to be a contribution or a detriment to the therapeutic process will depend on two factors. One is the analyst's willingness and capacity to bear the bad feelings that inevitably arise in the treatment interaction and to process them in the patient's best interest. The other is the extent to which the analyst is able to contact and put into words, with a decreasing sense of accompanying risk, everything he or she might think and feel that might be likely to give rise to such bad feelings" (p. 324).

References

Bangor University. (2012). Psychologists reveal how emotion can shut down high-level mental processes without our knowledge. *Medicalxpress* (online news letter, June 2012).

Blizard, R. A. (2001). Masochistic and sadistic ego states: Dissociative solutions in the dilemma of attachment to an abusive caregiver. *Journal of Trauma & Dissociation*, 2, 37–58.

Bromberg, P. M. (1998). *Standing in the spaces: Essays on clinical process, trauma, and dissociation*. Hillsdale, NJ: The Analytic Press.

Bromberg, P. M. (2006) "Ev'ry Time We Say Goodbye, I Die a Little ...": Commentary on Holly Levenkron's "Love (and Hate) with the Proper Stranger". *Psychoanalytic Inquiry*, 26, 182–201.

Bromberg, P. M. (2012). Credo. *Psychoanalytic Dialogues*, *22*, 273–278.

Epstein, L. (1984). An interpersonal-object relations perspective on working with destructive aggression. *Contemporary Psychoanalysis*, *20*, 651–662.

Epstein, L. (1999). The analyst's "Bad-Analyst Feelings." *Contemporary Psychoanalysis*, *35*, 311–325.

Guntrip, H. (1971). *Psychoanalytic theory, therapy, and the self*. New York, NY: Basic Books.

Liotti, G. (2004). Trauma, dissociation, and disorganized attachment: Three strands of a single braid. *Psychotherapy: Theory, Research, Practice, Training*, *41*, 472–486.

Mitchell, S. A. (1998). Aggression and the endangered self. *Psychoanalytic Inquiry*, *18*, 21–30.

Mitchell, S. A. (2000). Intersubjectivity: Between expressiveness and restraint in the analytic relationship. In *Relationality: From attachment to intersubjectivity* (pp. 125–146). Hillsdale, NJ: The Analytic Press.

Pizer, B. (2000). The therapist's routine consultations: A necessary window in the treatment frame. *Psychoanalytic Dialogues*, *10*, 197–207.

Pizer, B. (2003). When the crunch is a (k)not: A crimp in relational dialogue. *Psychoanalytic Dialogues*, *13*, 171–192.

Pizer, S. A. (1992). The negotiation of paradox in the analytic process. *Psychoanalytic Dialogues*, *2*, 215–240.

Russell, P. L. (1996). Process with involvement: The interpretation of affect. In L. E. Lifson (Ed.), *Understanding therapeutic action: Psychodynamic concepts of cure* (pp. 201–216). Hillsdale, NJ: The Analytic Press.

Russell, P. L. (2006a). The compulsion to repeat. *Smith College Studies in Social Work*, *76*, 33–49. (Original work published 1987)

Russell, P. L. (2006b). The negotiation of affect. *Contemporary Psychoanalysis*, *42*, 621–636. (Original work published 1976)

Russell, P. L. (2006c). The role of loss in the repetition compulsion. *Smith College Studies in Social Work*, *76*, 85–98. (Original work published 1988)

Russell, P. L. (2006d). The theory of the crunch. *Smith College Studies in Social Work*, *76*, 9–21. (Original work published 1975)

Russell, P. L. (2006e). Trauma, repetition, and affect. *Contemporary Psychoanalysis*, *42*, 601–620.

Stern, D. B. (1997). *Unformulated experience: From dissociation to imagination in psychoanalysis*. Hillsdale, NJ: The Analytic Press.

Stern, D. B. (2010). *Partners in thought*. New York, NY: Routledge.

Winnicott, D. W. (1990/1971). *Playing and reality*. New York, NY: Basic Books.

Wu, Y. J., & Thierry, G. (2012). How reading in a second language protects your heart. *The Journal of Neuroscience*, *32*, 6485–6489.

Reverie

Sometimes People Have to

Sometimes people have to do it over—but the second time it feels like work. Or

too much risk.

Knowing *that* you want

Knowing *what* you want

Getting what you want

And it is so fragile. Because for a while, when you don't get what you want, you want to take it personally—and the whole process is in danger of undoing, i.e.,

I shouldn't have wanted it, and/or

I wanted the wrong thing, and/or

I didn't want what I wanted badly enough, or

I NEVER WANTED IT IN THE FIRST PLACE!

Then you are at square one all over again.

I'm not looking for anything!

DOI: 10.4324/9781032666303-16

Maintaining Analytic Liveliness
"The Fire and the Fuel" of Growth and Change[1]

Introducing Aaren Kahn

When a patient lets me know he has changed his first name, I don't say anything right away, but I take notice. And when you stop to think about it, you realize I'm not saying very much about my own prescience or patience because, after all, it was Aaren who gave me the notice. Patients take their own sweet time to let you in on personal things. But the particular point I want to make here is that even *after* Aaren told me about this name change (on the day I handed him his first bill), I didn't know how to think about it. Often I would just forget. . .

Aaren Kahn was born and named Aaron Kahn. He still *is* Aaren Kahn. His secret is hidden in the spelling. Aaren spells himself with an *e*—Aaren Kahn—instead of the *o* he was born with—Aaron Kahn. Now if it was simply a matter of hiding his ethnicity, he could have worked on his last name instead; removed the *h*, added an *e*, and turned himself into Aaron Kane. But that wasn't the crux of what he decided to do. To my ear, and I imagine everybody else's, Aaren Kahn is still Aaron Kahn. So what's my story?

Maybe I should begin with a brief portrait of how I view this man: middle height, middle aged, a hidden sweetness somewhere, but nothing particular to say about his looks except in those sudden, open moments when he breaks into the most remarkable smile because of a pun he makes—original and ridiculously funny!

And I mustn't forget to mention this nonverbal quirk that I've grown so accustomed to, it barely registers on my perceptual map. You might call it a tick of some sort, or now that I come to think of it, a rhythmic ticking like

DOI: 10.4324/9781032666303-17

a metronome. It's a syncopating gesture Aaren makes when he is working through an idea or trying to recapture some vague remembrance. He'll tilt his head up, maybe focus on what's coming out of him, and his right arm raises at the elbow, with pointer and middle finger slightly crooked, the hand conducts a formulation back and forth to accompany whatever it might be that can or cannot be said.

Aaren, father of three—Rachel, Benjamin, and Sarah—married a psychologist, which may account for the large store of quotes and facts he holds about analytic theorists and theories. Perhaps his extensive knowledge of psychology (along with other esoteric subjects) contributes to his success as a lawyer, but who knows? Maybe his hunger for every kind of information relates to his favorite grandfather, who owned a grocery around the corner and knew all the items of his varied inventory in his head by heart! Only Aaren's Bubbe let him handle the long-poled grocery grabber that he rode like a horse around the town in Bubbe's game of search and grab the Kellogg's Crunch. Or maybe Aaren's endless quest for intellectual erudition helps defend against depression over having dropped his natural musical gifts and the pursuit of a life-long wish to play his violin in a national orchestra.

Not that he should change his profession or anything—after all, he and a group of friends have formed a little quartet, and they do play together when they find the time. But I have have said to Aaren on more than one occasion that I thought his giving up his dream of a musical career sits inside him like an ungrieved stone that puts a barrier between himself and feeling free with other people. Little did I know, when we began together, the full extent of the inertial drag of loss on this man's living. But I am getting ahead of myself.

Before going on about Aaren and me, I need to bring up some unavoidable truths about the telling. We need to keep reminding ourselves—or I do, anyway—that interactions in the consulting room unfold before we actually realize what is experienced within and between the two persons involved. We may be forming an impression that's attached to an idea, but there is nothing reliable to count on in the moment. *Experiencing* precedes whatever theoretical view we have about what happened. Naturally, we can't avoid our preconceptions, nor should we even try. But it helps me to bear in mind that whatever working assumption I pick up from the past necessarily narrows the field of present experiencing. That's just how it is. Anyway, when I do come around to putting my theory together with clinical narrative, or even the narrative with a theory in order to tell it to my colleagues, you have to know I am doing a kind of piecemeal, biased, backward job. However I might end up telling you my narrative, much of the story remains as silently out of sight as the story of Aaren Kahn, born Aaron Kahn, is Aaren Kahn.

For example, Aaren Kahn has come to my home office for over ten years, beginning in the summer of 1996. He soon became my first appointment of the morning. Always he arrives early and always with a book. On his days, initially, for some unthinkable reason, I have left the door between my office and the waiting room open—allowing Aaren the freedom to come in and sit on my couch to read before I arrive. Some place in my awareness, I must have recognized the absolute necessity for Aaren to prepare himself in my space in this particular way before we could attempt to be with one another. Not that he hadn't *already told me* that he always carried a book around, a book chosen from the latest stack picked up at the library. He *told me* that waiting at the train station to go to work he reads, riding the train he reads, sitting on a stool in the department store while his youngest daughter, Sarah, shops, Aaren reads. He "has to do it" is all that he can say. I "knew" this to be a fact, but that is not the way I took it to heart.

The reason I can grasp Aaren's need to sit in my space with a book before he can look up and return my greeting is because it happened in a process of awareness operating well ahead of my carrying it forward as an explicit bit of felt meaning. I can refer to an aspect of it now because of that experience one morning, when unmindful of the clock, I walked into my office fifteen minutes early. Shocked to discover my patient already well ensconced and comfortably in his place, I hastily excused myself and retreated. Can you imagine that! *Retreated*. From my own office! Almost stealthily, I moved back into my home quarters, biding my time until a few minutes before the appointed hour.

In this moment, I'm not exactly sure why I felt so ashamed about leaving my door open and then having backed off like that. Is it really ashamed that I was feeling? Kind of stupid. Territorial even.

The body's sense of wishing to hide was familiarly apparent, and I could talk about that—*but what matters more in this moment is to emphasize that in relating my story or in the telling of any clinical case, we must continuously try to inquire into how our theories—like Aaren's unexamined secrets—have the power to potentiate or wall us off from moving feelings forward in some meaningful direction.*

As therapists, we need to keep checking the assumptions that we make and to let them go the minute we learn otherwise. For example, initially, I see Aaren as somewhat insensitive, self-involved, and certainly controlling. But on that day that I came back into my office—sheepishly and a tinge resentful—Aaren looked up from his book and spoke as if he'd read my mind.

"I stopped feeling emotional years ago," he told me.

It's not unusual, I think, to receive more data about a person's life and living in the very first meeting or even in the first month of meetings, before anybody really knows what's going on—before expectations and self-consciousness set in.

"I've always had a problem with connection. I really like my kids but it makes me anxious. It bothers me that I don't know how to connect with them."

From what I understood so far, Aaren's growing up at home an only child was disrupted by random slaps and accusations, on the one hand, and smoothed over by what he called "overindulgence," on the other. "I never had to do a dish," he said. "but then again, my mother hardly ever paid attention. She was either watching soap operas or talking to her mother on the phone."

"Your grandfather," I said, "was that your father's father? What about him, your father I mean?"

"Dad pretty much adored me," Aaren commented offhandedly. "He took me to concerts but. . . " His voice broke off.

"Can you go on with that?"

"I remember he took me at a very young age. We'd be sitting there in the row, and he'd whisper in my ear that I should just touch his shoulder when I'd had enough. But. . . "

"Go with that," I urged.

"There was never a time I didn't know my father lived the life he didn't get to have by living it through me. I don't want to be like that with my kids. I don't want to be like either one of my parents. So I have trouble connecting."

"I don't quite get what you mean, Aaren, about your father living through you."

Briefly, Aaren sketched an image of "no love lost" between his parents: a lot of disdain and no end of screaming. Chaos. Then at night when Aaren was finally able to turn off his light for sleep, his father would come into the darkened room, stand by the bed, and probe for all the details of Aaren's day. "Let's recapitulate," his father would say.

"And what would you say?"

"Oh, come off it, Dad!" Aaren waved us both away.

I have no idea what Aaren read into my face, if anything; or what, if anything I felt. I do know that this was the last continuous conversation I would have with Aaren Kahn for a long, long time. It was Aaren who brought that session to a close.

"I stopped feeling emotional years ago," he warned. "My mother was a screamer and the chaos overwhelms me."

The Paradox of Theory and Experiencing

Holding theoretical considerations while maintaining analytic liveliness may constitute a paradox that we have to deal with from the start. Speaking for myself, resonant theories serve as essential tools when I connect them with my current experiencing in the moment. I don't mean to say that my sense of an arrangement of particular character traits won't call to mind a theorist I've read. In the initial phases of being with Aaren, I might well have glanced over to my bookshelf at the faded, once-blue dust jacket of a book containing a collection of Harry Guntrip's papers about schizoid phenomena. I might even have paused to wonder about Aaren's insurance diagnosis and whether or not I'd ever put schizoid or avoidant personality on a form because a metronome is not the music of experiencing.

A resonant theory works the other way around. You've been sitting with a person for a period of time, and then something nags at you that is unfamiliar. You can't quite recognize the thing. But if you focus on the ambiguity, if you attend to it, refer to it within yourself, you get a kind of nonverbal sense. After a while, you find a word or a phrase that may or may not match up with this sense, and you keep on going until you feel like you've got it. Often it is at this point that a resonant theory arrives in your head full-blown; *it* connects to *you* like a sudden unexpected guest who puts the whole thing in perspective.

Actually, I'm talking about a theory of theory that doesn't belong exclusively to any particular psychoanalytic school of thought. It is an intrapsychic theory that is ultimately facilitated by an intersubjective process that Eugene Gendlin (1964, 1981, 2007) has explicated. "Focusing" is an individual, one-person process, a "felt process" in which some "implicit meaning" interacts with some other feeling, meaning, or event and moves toward "symbolic completion."

But "symbolic completion" does not imply arrival at some dead-end theoretical street. One thing leads to another ("referent movement") and, as Gendlin (1964) emphasizes, the "implicit or felt datum of experiencing is a sensing of body life" (p. 11). Once we carry that datum forward and connect it to explicit meaning, we are no longer stuck with the theoretical concept hanging off by itself, but rather there is "an *interaction* between felt meaning and symbols or events" (p. 12). With the help of theory, something new may open up for us. Some fresh energy. No matter how humiliating or distressing the secret that we have hidden away may be, there is something relieving about bringing it into awareness. Felt datum allows us to experience a coming into being in the present time as well as the potential for carrying forward this felt datum toward a future something else.

I want to say again that this is a process that happens inside one person. Where it begins, and where and how it moves forward depends a good deal on that person's growth and development in the context of others. We know that by now. It is the paradox outlined by Winnicott (1965/1958) in his description of a capacity that is contingent on "the experience of being alone while someone else is present" (p. 30), in a reliable and unimpinging way.

Within any given analytic hour, the patient may be alone in the presence of the analyst and also together in transitional space, sometimes still, sometimes at work or play. The analyst and her resonant theories may do likewise, with the analyst forming an internal relationship with her resonant theories that is reliable and unimpinging, with theory serving in the wings of experiencing "represented for the moment by a general atmosphere in the immediate environment" (Winnicott, 1965/1958, p. 30) or perhaps only by a sensitivity, a vulnerability, or an analytic attitude.

As a practicing Relational analyst, I have become progressively aware of two intersecting vulnerabilities of my own. Even though my work has always been centered in the body-mind connection, even though I *know* that the expression of emotion without meaning is as hollow as an unfelt idea, I notice these moments when I find myself off balance, leaning too far over from experience into the soup of feeling or defensively removed by the pull of heady intellectual constructs. Either way, this vulnerability is about losing balance and going too far in one direction or another.

Then there is the other, linking vulnerability that signals me inside like the twang of a tightrope between guilt and shame. It happens when I am passionately headed off in one direction or another with somebody, and I let go of the dialectic that I take such pride in, the tension that defines the very essence of relationality. It's the too-late tremble in my stomach that tells me I have privileged intersubjectivity at the cost of disattending to the intrapsychic process. What makes me do that? I wonder. A kind of single-minded, universal tendency in all of us, perhaps, that leaves us stranded in either direction on a one-way street. For Aaren Kahn it's more like a cul-de-sac. I experience him racing around at breakneck speed, trying to disappear and then suddenly interrupting the spin to alter course. No transition. I imagine that underneath his feverish activity of words, he's hiding out. "Being with people," he says, "is exhausting most of the time."

The Firewall

"I read in this book review," Aaren's fingers are conducting, "where the author is a pianist who lost her music when she remembered what happened to her as a child."

"Yes," I respond. "The book is called *Memory Slips*, I think." The title brings his attention to a dream from last night.

> *My mother was on trial for murder. I was distant. . .in the back of the courtroom. Then I figured she'd probably go to jail for life and I'd never see her again. I should go up and hold her hand. I started to go down to her and then I woke up.*

Sitting with Aaren—rarely does he choose to lie down on my couch, I inadvertently mirror his kind of sucking in of a sigh. He turns away. By now having told myself a thousand times to *back off*, I once again experienced an internal wash of shame. I am blushing for having moved in too close. Maybe then I also turn away. Maybe Aaren caught me doing that, which is why he called me back by explaining that he *does* want to be understood but *not* made aware of something that he doesn't know.

Without skipping a beat, he points to the brocaded box on my windowsill and asks me what is in it.

"You can look and see," I say.

"What's in it??"

I reach over and pick up the box. "I was given these," I tell him, opening the box by its hinge and showing him the two shiny silver spheres—about the size of marbles—that are neatly housed inside. "They are called Chinese exercise balls," I go on to say, "and you're supposed to roll them around in your palm in a certain way so that they touch all your pressure points and, supposedly, it gets you to relax." I close the box and place it back on the sill.

Aaren reaches over and picks it up. Extracting the silver balls and placing the box on the flat of his book, he begins to roll the balls around his palm until he finds a rhythm that seems to suit him.

As he becomes entranced by this new task, another verbal process is set in motion.

"My mother told me that she had a life, before she had a son."

"Oh, dear," is all that my surprise can muster. On my side, I think that my implicit recognition of a felt sense of shame—the blush—might have been communicated in such a way that Aaren could move beyond his own avoidant experience with some relief. As I sit there continuing to wonder why in Aaren's bland company, I so hastily disown myself, and as I once again picture the morning that I came upon him by surprise and literally disappeared, Aaren offers up another clue.

"The son," he says flatly, "the first one that my mother had. That wasn't me."

"Oh!" Another shock. "I thought you were an only child."

"I am. The first Aaron died the day after he was born."

I'm not exactly sure when Aaren told me that he was named after the dead baby. I can't seem to find the information in my notes where it lies hidden. Now I realize that I "forgot" or kept it out of my experience for a long time after that. Something told me I needed to leave it alone.

"So many things in my life that I did that I'm ashamed of," he was telling me, "that I just shed my skin of them."

I remember saying, "Just the skin?"

No answer.

"You crawl away from those things but you take yourself with you."

I have no idea how I got away with that. But I remember Aaren telling me that he was given the same Hebrew name as his brother, Aaron Menachem Kahn. I also remember that Aaren wondered if his mother hated him for replacing the first one. And suddenly it came to him, "Maybe that's why my Dad was so overprotective!" So Aaren simply dropped his middle name, as he would do with other legacies of memory, and changed the spelling of his first.

I couldn't hold on to the knowledge myself. Despite the initial impact of Aaren's revelations, they seemed to fall away from my experiencing without the slightest evidence of having made a mark. Aaren Kahn, devoid. Aaren Kahn, possessor of an invisible magic trick that suddenly disrupted liveliness and blanked associations. I could not hold on to things. Neither bored nor drowsy, I could find no compass point in the whiteout of my mind, and there was too much buzzing in my body. Nothing coalesced. Restless may be more to the point. I was vigilant to catch the slightest intimation of alarm.

Aaren, for a number of years to come, controlled our space. Not that he wouldn't tell me things from time to time, little "shocks" outside of the endlessly driven ribbons of informative material that filled the interstices between us, strings of facts that passed for conversation. What I mean is, Aaren would tell me things, important things, deep things, but they seemed to come from nowhere and then get banished from between us. Now I could almost see the process of his words fading away like Cheshire cats and vanishing in thin air. A lack of continuity is what it was. We had no scaffolding on which to build a narrative for future growth.

Once I heard the phrase "I feel like a monster." It arrived out of the blue while Aaren flipped the pages of his book or fiddled with some object he had picked off my widowsill to play with. Occasionally, if I remembered to look elsewhere, a dream would follow.

I dreamed I was eating at a cannibal feast. It was wonderful food. But I knew when I was finished, I would be eaten.

Relating, he repeatedly insisted, was much too dangerous. He lets me in on an old secret. He has erected a "firewall" to hide behind. "Even though I get so lonely there," he says, "it keeps me safe."

"Safe?" as if I hadn't heard.

"My firewall is up."

Experiencing Ambiguity and State Shifts

Internally, I work to shake away a vacuous blocking that threatens to suck the life and music out of both of us. For a while, I would seek to be impressed by the huge amount of information that he has mastered. I know that for a while I even tried to memorize these facts to see what would happen if I passed them back in some new context, but gradually I felt myself go dry—imprisoned by the logic and the linearity of repetitive intellectual patterns that I couldn't help but imagine were tying us both up behind that firewall.

I seem to have lost the resources of wondering and inquiry. What comes into my mind is a sonnet by Robert Lowell (2003). I want to read it to him but I don't. It begins:

> Say life is the one-way trip, the one-way flight,
> say this without hysterical undertones—
> then you could say you stood in the cold light of science,
> seeing as you are seen, espoused to fact.

(p. 470)

"What, if anything, do I want," Aaren muses. "*I want to know things that I don't know before anyone else can tell me*. My parents always told me who I was and how I felt. They said that I was smarter than the other kids, and musical, and that was why the kids would bully me. I was above them." Aaren is stretching his neck. "Didn't feel like that to me," he adds.

"Were you afraid," I say offhandedly, "you afraid of the bullies?"

"I wake up anxious, in a panic. I broke a toy when I was a kid and my mother told me I was destructive and selfish. That's just what she said. I'm selfish, destructive. And smart. That's me."

Period. End of story. My question crept under the radar of our firewall and that was it. I could not speak to the odd, creeping terror that emerged between us. I felt paralyzed. But in the middle of that terror, I sensed something incredibly sweet and almost newborn about this man, and I wanted to reach out to him, to hold his frightened-child face in my hands, and yet he had me paralyzed. The bitter words of Robert Lowell (2003) continue in my head:

> Strange, life is both the fire and fuel; and we
> the animals and objects, must be here
> without striking a spark of evidence
> that anything that ever stopped living
> ever falls back into living when life stops.

(p. 470)

"That's it!" I say to myself. "He won't strike a spark of evidence!" But then it occurs to me that Lowell got it backward. You start with fuel to make a fire, and eventually, the fire goes out. You've run out of fuel, and that's the end of that. I'm sounding just like Aaren. End of story.

One day, and who knows why, Aaren presented another dream. He had gone to China, looking to find a rare and ancient extinct fish. I asked him what kind of a fish. "A Coelacanth," he answered, pronouncing it S-E-A-L-Acanth, for clarification. I asked if he could tell me about this fish and anything more about the dream. "It took place in a museum in China and the Coelacanth was floating in the water. . . hovering, down at the bottom of a glass beaker. A murky muddy icky fish, and I didn't know if it was dead or alive."

I could not form a question in my mind. That night, I googled the thing. I learned that Coelacanths "are the only living species known to have a functional *intracranial* joint, which almost completely separates the front and back halves of the *skull* internally. Flexure at this joint may aid in the consumption of large prey by the use of suction." Coelacanths are also mucilaginous; "their scales release mucus and their bodies exude oil. . . makes the fish almost inedible unless dried and salted." No more, no more. Dried and salted. I believe Aaren at one point asked me if I'd like to try and eat one.

At this point, you may have made all the connections that you need between your preferred theory and our unfolding story to understand at least one strand of the secrets held by Aaren Kahn. But let me be clear that I return to this story as my way of carrying fragments forward toward symbolic completion "*after backwards*" you might say. For Aaren and me, I am now searching for aspects of felt data that, at the time, I stopped referring to, felt meanings that I kept under wraps, dissociated you might say, for Aaren's safety as well as mine.

I mean, what good does it do to enter into Aaren's life someplace before the two of us can go there together in awareness? He *already told us that*! And for me to know I think I know a some "thing" living inside Aaren without telling him is adding one more secret to the chaos or the firewall. I sense myself treading in dangerous territory.

These are the times that I seek solace from company with a favorite theorist of mine. The citation that I use here arrives long after Aaren's murky fish, but it is the one that comes alive for me now upon this writing. "Psychological self-continuity," Bromberg (2006) writes,

> plays a role that is as central for survival of a member of the human species as biological self-continuity is for lower forms of life. When

self-continuity seems threatened, the mind adaptationally extends its reach beyond the moment by turning future into a version of past danger.... The linear experience of time is collapsed into itself as a protective device, producing relative amnesia for perceptual memory of past trauma but leaving bodily and affective memory intact, often horrifyingly intact.

(pp. 4, 5)

It puzzles me the way that Aaren's mother prompted, I imagine, by her unarticulated sense of loss and failure, would love him one minute and beat him up the next without, according to Aaren, the slightest provocation. She didn't drink. I realize something is still missing from his story. Where his father was. Again, I would not suggest that Aaren "recapitulate."

As Bromberg (2006) continues: "This time condensation supports the early warning system by freezing the person's image of the future and of the present into replicas of the past" (p. 5).

This sort of stoppage or blockage of ongoing interactive processes—both within and between participants in the consulting room, curtailment of the implicit function of felt experiencing—is what Gendlin (1964) calls "structure bound," or, similar to Bromberg, relating in "frozen wholes" whose meaning originates in an unremembered past.

Herein lies a set of critical clinical questions. How to be with the dead self-state in another that neither violates the other nor annihilates the self? How do we locate felt experiencing within ourselves when experiencing within the other is adamantly denied or when it is specifically requested that we do not know what we might know before the other finds it in himself? How, in this blocked self-state, do we be with all of what is and is not happening while still keeping track of who is who in the interaction? At what moment do we discover that we have lost touch with the thread that may have gone lax but holds us together in a grip we are too numb to grasp in understanding?

Now in retrospect, I move into a moment where I let the thread go lax in my concern with Aaren. It felt unbearable to me. So I broke off my connection to the crazy coexistence of paralysis and maternal passion by turning to an argument with Robert Lowell. Numb to Aaren, my own predicament, and the poet's nonlinear dynamic metaphor of life as "fire and fuel," I gave up on the dialectic, moved over to my mind, and there I let the whole thing drop.

Might this be the universal human tendency that Lowell highlights in his sonnet's sad conclusion?

> There's a pale romance to the watchmaker God
> of Descartes and Paley; He drafted and installed
> us in the Apparatus. He loved to tinker;
> but having perfected what He had to do,
> stood off shrouded in his loneliness.

(p. 470)

Personally, I associate "the Apparatus" with an image of the incubator where I had been placed as a preemie in the first weeks of life. Certainly the opposite of how it must have been, I imagine my tiny person in the pitch-black dark, and I experience the retrospective horror of an abandoned self sealed off from contact.

Was it Aaren, then, who felt the challenge of my implicit sense of isolation? Did he feel it in the oxygen we breathed behind the firewall?

With no explicit sense of my preoccupation, and shortly after that, Aaren actually composed a poem of his own—written much in the arcane style of Robert Lowell—wordlessly handing it over for me to have. It is a poem, I'm ashamed to say, that utterly escaped my mind until I decided to look back and found it. Consider Aaren's last five lines:

> The force tied into you comes from the darkness
> And from the nonself that is not you.
> It's a poison that seeps into you, not from you.
> It is Antaeus:[2] Lift it to the sky
> And watch it lose its hold on you and die.

Adding to my shame, I never asked Aaren who Antaeus was. Whether or not he registered such analytic ignorance, a few months later he passed me another simpler verse. It is only in this very moment that I *feel* the deceptive irony in Aaren's title:

> Nursery Rhyme
> Sit in your corner
> Sit in your box
> Don't take off your shoes
> Don't take of your socks

I'm sitting in mine
But I know you're there
'Cause I feel your crying
Under my chair.

Tipping Points

The thing about reflection in hindsight is that dissociated past events become so meaningful when you experience the links in the relative safety of the present. You can connect the dots or forge new pathways between self-states and finally get the feeling of what was always there. But when the butterfly in Rio flits its wings, you are not yet aware of the hurricane about to happen in Miami. The tipping points that create the total context for the direction that experiencing will take have not yet emerged.

Looking back, I find so many clues that escaped my inquiry or wonder, like the identity of Antaeus—giant, bully, and son of Mother Earth, who slew all challengers until Hercules discovered the maternal secret of his power; like why it was that Aaren, only son but younger brother of the son who died, referred to Sarah as "the free child."

Also, over the last five years, I began to notice a shift in my behavior with Aaren. Rather than arriving promptly for our sessions (an inbred childhood habit born of fear), I started coming late without realizing it at first. In 2002, I write to myself that Aaren is pissed with me. Why else would he keep falling asleep in his sessions? Just sitting there, drowsing away.

"'Alone in the presence of another,'" Aaren quips, quoting Winnicott before he falls off to sleep. "I hope he realizes I don't disappear on him like that," I say to myself. *But what am I talking about?* What is it supposed to mean, my coming late?? And when he falls asleep, I remember a paper that Ogden (1988) wrote, "Misrecognitions and the Fear of Not Knowing." I picture Ogden, the analyst, sitting in a dead spot with his patient as he becomes aware of his *own detachment from himself!* In feeling that experience, Ogden is able to make reference to the felt experience of his patient's world.

Thus, Rephrasing Winnicott and others in this new context, Ogden traces the unconscious fear of not knowing and the modes of defense against such fears. The analyst dissociates or resorts to filling the space with the borrowed authority of his theories and expertise.

Thinking of Ogden, I begin to get back in touch with the ways in which the mantled intensity of Aaren's competing self-states–the bully and the bullied–mirror my own. And then I lose track of where, if any place, I am. As Ogden (1988) writes, "The patient," and, I might add, the analyst,

> is both mother and infant, both misrecognizing and misrecognized. In the context of this internal relationship, the patient [and analyst] experiences anxiety, alienation, and despair in connection with the feeling of not knowing what it is he feels or who, if anyone, he is.
>
> (p. 664)

In the next session, without a thought, I simply handed Aaren a copy of Ogden's paper. Imagine my surprise when, two sessions later, Aaren wordlessly brought it back to me. I note that he had taken his yellow highlighter and underlined the sentences and phrases that drew his attention and that he wanted me to see.

As I see it now, Aaren's quipping quote of Winnicott, "Alone in the presence of another" was a tipping point as were his poems and the process of highlighting in private his connections with me by way of Ogden's words. Hidden secrets placed into my hands.

Touched by this image, I experience a body sense of the "thing" that Winnicott was talking about, neither the impingement of an object parent nor the abandonment I felt inside the imagined darkness of an incubator. I ask myself what it feels like to me now—"the capacity to be alone." It feels like *rest*. Like a bugle playing "Taps" at night. "All is well, safely rest." What might it mean for Aaren to exist for a time without impingement, internalized by now, without interrupting himself or hiding out behind the firewall? I think about "alone *in the presence of another*," the paradoxical provision that creates a space for intrapsychic process alongside an available potential to interact and play.

Then all at once, I realize what was there all along. It's not that Aaren is unable to focus on his own experience. It's not that he can't formulate his thoughts. But in order to share them, he seems to require some ongoing and benign external source of movement to ensure safe passage along the way. I think of his conducting gestures. Yes, he interrupts himself. But there are times when I come in, in the morning, and see his eyes moving back and forth in rhythmic cadence as he scans the sentences delivered to him in the pages of a book. Do I detect a secret smile?

Bypassing some personal embarrassment, I allow into awareness of the variety of gadgets I have imported onto my windowsill, replacing, for example, the brocaded box of Chinese exercise balls with a hand-held trigger point massage tool called a Jacknobber. Formed in the shape of a child's jack but large enough to firmly grip with the fingers of one hand, Aaren would twirl one of its four wooden knobs on and off as he talked with me or brush it back and forth behind his neck and across his shoulder blades.

It came to me that Aaren, despite the shame he held inside the secrets of his childhood, had learned long ago in Bubbe's grocery store to grab hold of the experience of play and knew that he could ride it through in his imagination. That image brought me to the thought of a way that we might "go a stage further back," in Winnicott's (1965/1958, p. 30) words, while also moving forward.

Another tipping point: I turn over in my mind the idea of introducing Aaren to using the lightbar developed for a mode of processing experiencing called EMDR (Eye Movement Desensitization and Reprocessing)[3] that jumpstarts, so to speak, the patient's spontaneous associations.

Borrowing from EMDR

Over the next few years, Aaren and I have borrowed a technique from EMDR as an occasional resource for carrying forward the long-dormant implicit referents of his experiencing. The "Apparatus" of choice is a horizontal lightbar that I carry in from my office sunroom and set up at a comfortable distance opposite Aaren, who sits up on the couch. I sit to one side—in the wings of Aaren's experiencing—leaving him free and in control of the process, so that when he signals me, I click on the bright blue dots of light that stream back and forth across the bar—"just let your eyes follow the lights, Aaren, and see what comes up." His eyes move back and forth from right to left and left to right in a way that may simulate the eye movements of REM sleep. But in this event, Aaren does not sleep. Rather, he is awake and focused, the agent of his own processing, "alone in the presence of another."

For my purposes, I relate EMDR's processing of memory, feelings, and cognitions in experiential terms, comparing it with Gendlin's (1964) notions of growth and change. In his words:

As implicitly functioning felt meanings are *carried forward* and processing is *reconstituted* and made more immediate in manner, there is a constant change in "content." As referent movement occurs, both symbolization and direct referent change. There is a sequence of successive "contents." Sometimes these successive contents are said to "emerge" as if they had always been there, or as if the final basic content is now finally revealed. But I prefer to call this *content mutation*. It is not a change only in how one interprets but, rather, a change both in feeling and in symbols. The contents change because the process is being *newly completed and reconstituted* by responses.

(p. 30)

I conclude with two living examples from our story.

Our Session with the Lightbar 1/31/06

This is the eleventh of our twelve sessions with the lightbar that were spread over two years.

Aaren: "I wonder what it would feel like if I had been a *genuine* younger brother, instead of a *fake* only child."

Barbara: "Go with that."

Aaren: "What did that feel like that this baby died? Was he in pain?"

Barbara: "Go with that."

Aaren muses over his three children—girl—boy—girl. "Sarah is the one who has an older brother. Is my relationship with Ben colored by this in some way?"

Barbara: "Go with that."

Aaren: "I started thinking about Ben. He's got a girlfriend, and I don't want him to marry her. A father usually feels that way about his daughter. Why do I feel like that with Ben?"

Barbara: "Go with that."

Aaren: "Like I don't want to lose him. Though I barely feel connected to him. I find it easier to talk with the girls. I don't know what he gets from me."

Barbara: "Go with that."

Aaren: "I have *three* kids, not one. They have a relationship with each other that I didn't have. I wished I did."

Barbara: "Go with that."

Aaren: "I wish I weren't so alone."

Barbara: "Go with that."

Aaren: "My kids. These kids, they turn into Lords of themselves."

Barbara: "Tell me what you mean."

Aaren: "That's from *Dante's Inferno*. Virgil says it in *Purgatory*. 'Lord of Yourself, I crown and Miter you!'"

Barbara: "Your kids. They are Lords of Themselves. And you?"

Aaren: "In some ways I am. In some ways, I'm lost. *I don't want my brother's legacy.*"

The content of Aaren's responses in this session newly reconstitutes the felt meaning of what once I could not understand, that is, his reference to Sarah as "the free child."

Session 1/8/07

Before my vacation.

Aaren: "Having to walk a tightrope for four weeks long. How will I get through it alone? Without a net. Like in high school, having to swim from one end of the pool to the other. I was scared that I couldn't. I don't really believe I couldn't. I'm strong enough to make it. I'm telling myself I can't make it. I know I can."

Barbara: "Go with that."

Aaren: "When my grandfather died, nobody coming to be with me. He went to the hospital and didn't come back. My dad told me he went to heaven and would come back in fifty years. He didn't."

Barbara: "And if your grandpa were still alive?"

Aaren: "He played with me. He taught me to spin coins." Aaren's voice becomes the voice of a small child. "I went in his store and drank soda."

Barbara: "Yes?"

Aaren: "I can still spin coins. Sitting in a chair in his house. A dish of sourballs. His name was Samuel. He had five kids named after him. Nephews. He very suddenly and unexpectedly died."

Barbara: "Go with that."

Aaren: "Something died in me. My father said he'd gone to heaven, and he'd come back fifty years."

I noted that Aaren had stopped processing. He was beginning to freeze. So I asked him to show me how he can spin a coin. He pulls a quarter from his pocket and attempts the feat, using the marble cube table beside the couch. The coin falls flat. I imagine that the surface of the marble is too slippery. He tries again and fails.

"Too slippery," I say, asking for permission to bring over the little wooden table that sits next to my analytic chair. He nods assent but continues with the coin on marble.

"Can't work, Aaren, really, I don't think." Then Aaren turns to the wooden table now sitting where I have placed it in front of him. I hold my breath. The coin *spins*. It spins and spins until it wobbles to a halt. He does it again. And once again. We both laugh, triumphant. Once again he spins the coin.

Aaren says, "When Grandpa died, my world changed." He continues with the spinning. "Grandma would always choke up." Then he stops.

"You bring him alive," I say, "a good man to remember." And after a moment, feeling it was safe, I dare to say, "Your Grandpa was alive. Your brother was dead."

"Yes," says Aaren. And now more forcefully, "*You can't compete with a dead baby*!!"

"But here's the thing," I say to Aaren, handing him his coin from the table in case he might wish to give it another spin. "You have your Grandpa inside too."

Notes

1 A version of this chapter was delivered in 2007 at the Spring Meeting of Division 39 of The American Psychological Association, Toronto, Canada.
2 Antaeus was a giant in classical history, whose strength was invincible, challenging all comers to a wrestling match that he always won (slaughtering his victims) until he met Hercules. Each time Hercules threw Antaeus to the ground, Antaeus revived... until Hercules uncovered his secret. Antaeus' mother was Gaia (earth mother), who provided the source of his strength. So Hercules held the giant aloft until all his power drained away.
3 Francine Shapiro's EMDR, developed more than thirty years ago, is an integrated therapy that has eight phases, the most well known of which involves the processing of traumatic feelings, memories, and beliefs with the use of bilateral stimulation. While EMDR is a complete, stand-alone therapy, its full protocol can also be incorporated into other therapeutic frames. EMDRIA is the international association that certifies trained EMDR therapists.

References

Bromberg, P. L (2006). *Awakening the dreamer: Clinical journeys*. Mahwah, NJ: The Analytic Press.

Cutting, L. C. (1997). *Memory slips: A memoir of music and healing*. Mahwah, NJ: The Analytic Press.

Gendlin, E. T. (1964). A theory of personality change. In P. Worchel & D. Byrne (Eds.), *Personality change* (pp. 100–148). New York: John Wiley and Sons.

Gendlin, E. T. (1981). *Focusing*. New York, NY: Bantam Books.

Gendlin, E. T. (2007, June 23). Focusing: The body speaks from the inside. Presented at the 18th Annual International Trauma Conference, Psychological Trauma: Neuroscience, Attachment and Therapeutic Interventions. Boston, MA.

Lowell, R. (2003). *Watchmaker God. Collected poems of Robert Lowell*. New York, NY: Farrar, Straus and Giroux.

Ogden, T. H. (1988). Misrecognitions and the fear of not knowing. *Psychoanalytic Quarterly*, *57*, 643–666.

Winnicott, D. W. (1965/1958). The capacity to be alone. In *The Maturation Process and the Facilitating Environment* (pp. 29–36). New York, NY: International Universities Press.

Reverie

To Tell the Truth

To tell the truth, I feel like someone who has been battered. I know I'm not crazy, but what I mean to say is that my dissociation is so powerful and such a way to survive my life that it *feels* like craziness. At least I recognize that feeling for what it is.

Besides feeling creepy, dissociation feels like not being able to get to something I know very well is right at my fingertips, but I automatically dissociate to not feel.

But I feel like someone who has been battered even though I may be the batterer.

DOI: 10.4324/9781032666303-18

Chapter 12

"Trauma, Dissociation, and Disorganized Attachment"

A Clinical Collage Engaging Giovanni Liotti's Work[1]

An Image of Claire and Me

When my patient was forty-five and I was seventy, we played the game of searching out a name for her that I could use as I set out to tell the story of our work. It seemed to both of us a mischievous activity that would, to our surprise, temporarily break the current spell of unaccountable despair. She sat beside me on the couch leaning against the plastered-over hole in the wall through which she had once long ago smashed her head and scanned the dismal horizon behind her eyes. Suddenly, she dove down inside herself and came back up victorious. It was as if she had caught a glistening silver fish. A wry, conspiratorial smile: "We will call me Claire!"

"Yes!" my thumbs-up reply.

The Transgenerational Transmission of Trauma: Dissociation and Disorganized Attachment

Claire was not yet fifteen that summer of 1978 when she first came to my office accompanied by her mother. Whether by accident or design, the girl waited outside for some little while, allowing Mrs. Claire to brief me before she took her turn. Mrs. Claire greeted me with an immediate flash of smile. An attractive woman impeccable in her cobalt-linen suit that set off her brilliant blue eyes, she comported herself to the nearest chair and gently subsided—still smiling—onto its seat. Mrs. Claire appeared competent, uneasy, perhaps shy.

"Tell me," I said, "how I can be of help?"

"Claire's natural father died seven years ago," she chirped. "Four years after that I married again." I detected a quaver in the high pitch of her disowned voice, as if she were speaking to me through a tube. It might

DOI: 10.4324/9781032666303-19

have been the pressure of courageous effort that beckoned me to like her. "My husband has a drinking problem," she pressed on, "and Claire harbors an intense dislike of him." Was it her voice or her spirit that broke at this moment? "I need to be more supportive of Claire, but not the middle person."

"I see," I said softly. And waited.

Mrs. Claire, her tone just around the corner from hysteria, bent her best effort to contribute to the task at hand. Yes, she's afraid she did suffer a general depression at the time of Claire's birth—her second child. In those days it never occurred to her that one had a choice about having children. Herself the only child of a cold, self-occupied, withholding woman, Mrs. Claire explained that in her ignorance she treated her own three offspring likewise. Now the reality of her pain rang true in her tone as she recalled an isolated childhood: "When I received dolls as gifts," she sighed, "I would take off their clothes, shut them away in a drawer, and never look at them again."

Giovanni Liotti (2004) stresses the clinical significance of "a major discovery in attachment research" that links "caregivers' unresolved memories of traumas or losses" with the development of early attachment disorganization in their children. (p. 473)

As for Claire's birth, "water broke in the morning, but I went about my business. Then she came fast, almost too fast, at five o'clock. But she was a quiet baby. Sucked her thumb in the playpen a lot."

I was a preemie myself, arriving in this world too fast. There's a photo of me in a playpen looking forlorn and sucking my thumb. I am also a second child. My parents, who fled from Hitler with their eldest just a toddler, claim to have conceived me on the day they set foot on American soil—back then the land of hope and freedom. But my mother could hardly speak English as she combed the supermarket aisles in search of cereal for her one-year-old. *"Gries,"* she pleaded in her native tongue—*gries*, the German word for what she desperately needed and could not obtain.

"What should I do? What should I say?"

Claire seemed relaxed when she came into the office and took her mother's place. She seemed taller and probably less frail than her mother, though who could tell from the slouch of sweaters that she wore both under and over her overalls. Nevertheless, I saw in Claire's face and eyes a delicate fawn, and she moved through space with the careless grace of a Botticelli Venus that shone through the many layers of her hidden selves.

Claire spoke lucidly on that first day, and little did we know that she would soon spend six months of twice-a-week therapy almost entirely mute. And we also didn't know that once her conversation would resume, she would speak to me either in gibberish or rather fluent German. She told me that she had no English.

"*Ich weiss es nicht.* [I do not know.] *Ich weiss es nicht.*"

From Liotti (2004):

Dissociation is usually defined as a deficit of the integrative functions of memory, consciousness, and identity and is often related to traumatic experiences and traumatic memories. (p. 473)

Here I was, newly engaged in my second career, and hardly experienced. I was soon to learn that I committed enough errors to fill the volumes of Claire's journals, journals that I gingerly suggested we could exchange each week during her silence for my written comments in the margins. Whereas her mother was shy, Claire was intensely private. Guarded. (I was not permitted to address her by name or speak to her in the waiting room or anywhere else.) Her journals provided our first language.

Journal entry: "That lady I like, but she knows me not at all. She, I wish, I did not know. I did not know then what would happen. I wish I died when I was a day old. I am positive that the lady know nothing. Not her fault. It would have been the same with anyone. I just wish I could get away from her. But she is my breathing at all."

Indeed, breathing was just about all that I could offer, along with the ambiguous messages delivered from my heart and reading her diary of rage.

Journal entry: "She is like an awkward bystander at a crisis—pleading (except she doesn't plead because she doesn't see the situation) 'what should I do, what should I say?' Then they just stand there. I KNOW I make it impossible but I just wish she weren't so weak and empty handed and we could find each other."

Liotti (2004) emphasizes:

The dissociative power of this subtle type of trauma, betrayal from a not otherwise maltreating attachment figure, is readily explained by attachment theory. Forced by the inborn propensity to preserve the attachment relationship and trust the caregiver, when a parent denies the very existence of abuse perpetuated by another member of the family (or by a person outside the family), the abused child may collude with the parent's denial and dissociate the traumatic memory (Bowlby, 1998; Freyd, 1997). (p. 475)

Once we began to communicate in German, both of us sitting under the hot tent of a blanket so Claire would not be disturbed by the passage of air over her skin, my own young memories of the priest on Fire Island and my silent refugee mother floated back into our atmosphere. She could not know, could not know.

Several years later—journal entries and tent conversations lost to consciousness, perhaps dissociated—Claire called me from a phone booth in the nearby movie house where she held a summer job before her first year of college. She informed me that since she'd soon be dead, she wasn't coming for her two-o'clock hour this afternoon. With hardly a thought, I marched myself down to the movie house. It must have been between shows because the lobby was filled with patrons milling about. Claire was sitting inside the cashier cage.

"Claire," I hissed, "if you don't *promise me* this minute you'll be in my office at two o'clock this afternoon, I *promise you I will step back two feet from where I am standing in front of you, and I will holler Claire, CLAIRE, so loud that everybody and the whole world will hear me screaming out your name!*" She promised. At that, I spun around and marched back to my office.

And years later still, after nine hospitalizations (I held fast to whatever continuity I could through nightly phone exchanges and weekly visits), Claire hobbled from her car into my office barely able to walk. It seemed that she suffered some frightening dislocation of the spine so excruciating that even *she* could experience sensations of intense pain that broke through dissociation's barriers to feeling. (What an ironic index of our progress!) Over Claire's objections, I called her mother to come and get her. We were standing at the door when she arrived. Hurrying toward us, I saw for myself this most incredible look of anguish in mother's face. Was it anger or terror that had come to get Claire?

"What should I do," the mother pleaded, "What can I do?"

"*Fright without solution,*" a precursor to dissociation (Liotti, 2004, p. 477).

I watched Claire hobble into action, all the while soothing that lady. I watched the girl ease her aches into the mother's car. I heard her speak the words, "It's all right now mother, don't worry, I'll be okay."

Liotti (2004) from the work of Schore:

The right-brain system (connecting limbic emotional centers to the neo-cortex through the crossroad of the orbitofrontal cortex) that is involved in coping with emotional stressors develops along unfavorable lines in the face of chronic early relational traumas (Shore, 2001, 2002). This may be the neurological basis for the vulnerability to dissociative responses to traumatic stressors later in life. (p. 478)

"But I Cannot See and I Cannot Hear"

Claire and I worked hard to override various hospital consultants' cynical guarantee of a chronic patient's back-ward existence. (Although I don't hold the notion of "cure," the idea of "managing" a patient, or anyone else, is anathema to me.) In March of 1989, Claire entered and released herself from an institutional setting for the last time.[2]

Claire, a self-taught artist, musician, gifted photographer, creator of quilts and collages, has discovered concrete ways to put her selves and her worlds together. Today, stone by stone, she constructs the most extra-ordinary dry-laid walls—a metaphor indeed for the precise fitting together of petrified sections of sand (of dissociated life) without the mortar (the affect) to connect them. Claire has completed a ten-year course of analysis. She is now able to discern the triggers that send her flying into dissociation and can report them with considerable reflective functioning. But the sense of her self as "a human being among other human beings" (Kohut, 1984, p. 200) still remains unreal. Perhaps because in addition to her dissociation, *she cannot see and she cannot hear.* I have always believed this because, perhaps naively, I have placed my faith in Claire's reports of her personal (un) "reality" before there existed the BEAM Study in which she partici-pated in 1982 that showed bitemporal independent sharp-spike discharges and suggested more right-frontal than left-hemisphere difficulty. In 1990, with technology steadily improving, Claire undertook an Evoked Response Potential Test wherein her responses to aural and visual stimuli were meas-ured. In both areas, the data showed a nearly flat line.

"If I didn't know you better," declared the testing physician, "I'd say you were almost deaf and also suffered severe occipital damage." More specifically, Claire could take information into her senses up to the point where she could act on them without actually experiencing perception. Hence the working hypothesis: a brain abnormality in early development, possibly the result of severe early deprivation and subsequent traumatic episodes, underlay this anomalous functional pattern.

Liotti (2004) emphasizes that

> for the psychotherapy of complex trauma-related disorders … the patients' interpersonal difficulties should receive at least as much attention as their traumatic memories, their dissociative experiences, and their dissociative defenses.…Whenever there is a hint that a disorganized IWM [Internal Working Model] is guiding the patient's way of construing the therapeutic relationship, the correction of such a model should become a primary aim of the treatment. (pp. 482–483)

And further, that

> striving for safety and alliance within the therapeutic relationship should take precedence, both temporally and in the hierarchy of therapeutic aims throughout the treatment, over trauma work. (p. 483)

Claire and I sit on the couch and marvel. We have lived through her rages and my mistakes. Both of us have survived the transgenerational transmission of trauma, but actual traumas of commission did not take place within my family. We may assume that in hers they did. As a preemie, I was held and nurtured by an Irish nurse with instructions not to put me down. My father and grandma also nurtured me in those early years. When my mother at last revealed her truth, when I was the age that Claire is now, that her brother had sexually abused her in childhood, it was the greatest gift she could have given me—the gift of understanding something about myself. A gift that I could always use.

Where Claire was mute, raging, and dissociated, I was naive, assuaging, and dissociated. Whereas I recognize that I have failed my patient many times, I believe that I have never actually betrayed her. And somehow Claire has found it within herself to stick it out with me. She has moved from catatonia through dissociative nightmares and severe self-injury into a realm of selves held exquisitely almost together like her complex cubistic collages. Claire now maintains her own household, has a dog she cherishes, and has developed lasting intimate friendships. Although Claire is without a doubt more brilliant and more diversely gifted than I might ever be, unfortunately she cannot use these gifts to maximize her possibilities in the larger world. Our best hope, shared by us both, is that before I die, she will find a way to experience me that she can hold and remember. I see us both as women of courage and integrity.

For myself, I do not consider my integrity as virtue, but rather a transgenerational lifeline to survival. My directness of speech is often troublesome for friends and colleagues, but without this I am pulled back into helpless compliance. Far from a stranger to traumatic abuses, I would say that the taking of inordinate risks is the price I willingly pay in exchange for the isolation that sometimes can result when one is buried in self-recriminating shame.

Ten years ago, Claire requested that we celebrate our twenty-fifth "anniversary" by entering "the real world" for a dinner out at a "real restaurant" with my husband, who has served as a steady and safe male figure in the background of our clinical environment. We talked about this for a month and finally decided we could risk it. At the close of a quietly graceful and lightly conversational evening, I stood once more at the door with Claire before she would climb into her car. Suddenly, familiarly, her face switched. A blank stare.

"Who are you? Where am I?" she mumbled.

Holding her loosely by the shoulders to steady our connection, slowly, calmly, carefully, I replied. "My name is Barbara," I said, "and you are Claire. We are in the state of Massachusetts." I paused, allowing time for her to take that in. "We have just had a dinner, Claire, to celebrate because the two of us have been working very hard together *for twenty-five years*."

To which, with a return of that wry smile I have come to cherish, as if she had just caught a glistening silver fish, Claire ventured, "Can't you step it up a little?"

Notes

1 A version of this chapter was first presented in 2005 as an invited discussion of G. Liotti's "Trauma, Dissociation, and Disorganized Attachment: Three Strands of a Single Braid" for the International Association of Relational Psychoanalysis and Psychotherapy conference in Rome, Italy.

2 It has been so gratifying for Claire and me to discover, at last, a body of literature that braids together a substantive rationale for the ways in which we worked intuitively in the early years. For example, sharing the work with adjunct clinicians despite repeated early warnings that I was encouraging—God help us—a splitting of the transference rather than providing an opportunity for Claire to develop other attachments when she

felt too angry or too close to me for comfort, and for me a potential space should the pressure of her necessary and mutually acknowledged demands become too great to bear alone.

References

Liotti, G. (2004). Trauma, dissociation, and disorganized attachment: Three strands of a single braid. *Psychotherapy: Theory, Research, Practice, Training, 41*(4): 472–483.

Reverie
English Is My Mother's Second Language

English was my mother's second language, and she used it as an excuse. What I mean is, every time I'd ask her some private or personal thing that might draw us closer—like, what is French kissing and when is it okay to do, she'd say that she knew how to explain it in German, but she didn't have the English words to make it clear. And she'd tell me to go and ask my dad, who would certainly do a fine explanatory job.

I was in my forties before I learned about what happened to my mother growing up and that explains a lot. But I have to tell you about one exception to the rule of her sending me off to my dad. I remember, I was nine years old. I remember coming downstairs from my room to find my mother sitting on the loveseat darning socks. It had just become dusk, and she'd turned on the lamp. A whisp of her ash-blond hair fell across her forehead as she bent to her task.

"Mommy," I asked, "what is a perversion?"

Without even looking up, she replied, "Anything two people are doing and only one person enjoys."

I'll never forget it.

DOI: 10.4324/9781032666303-20

"Why Can't We Be Lovers?" When the Price of Love Is Loss of Love

Boundary Violations in a Clinical Context

A few days ago, I trashed the article I had mostly written. I couldn't bear it. That very night I had one of the worst nightmares I can ever remember …

The thing about such nightmares—I mean the kind that drenches you through your bedclothes and causes such a trembling, the odd part is that no matter how unique these nightmares may seem, the deeper themes that fuel them and even how the themes are symbolized turn out to be fairly common. Shame and a feeling of being overwhelmed, for example—like walking in a crowd of people and slowly noticing that you left home naked, or finding yourself unprepared for an exam in a required course you cannot remember taking, or forever trying to pack your bags while knowing your plane is about to depart, and so on. Do you think there is a case to be made for saying that most nightmares occur in slow motion?

But this nightmare has an added twist. It actually continued the following afternoon when the dream's dialogue I had completely lost (or dissociated) rose to consciousness, disrupting my senses in a way that I had never experienced before. That's what's memorable, I guess. Deep in the body where nightmares form, I can feel the rising intensity of alarm releasing into nervous laughter. How bizarre! Each time I hear the inane verbal threat embedded in my dream perpetrator's explicit warnings about how he plans to use me, soil me, I have to laugh. That's right. The words that come out of his mouth are so stupid! It's so embarrassing that laughing is all that's left. Sorry. And the damn dream wants to hang on. I cannot get rid of it. Maybe it's waiting for me to say the things out loud, tell you the embarrassing dialogue, relate the narrative of what my mind had made. But not yet. Not yet.

Let me attend to the main theme of this article first. Okay? Boundary Violations in a Clinical Context. What might be useful for me to say to

DOI: 10.4324/9781032666303-21

you from my personal experience of violation in my first analysis? And by the way, how do we make sense of the fact that telling that story feels less embarrassing than the silly nightmare dream did? Is that not strange?

The violation by my analyst occurred so long ago I should be over it already. Right? I am. I think, I thought, I mean, I thought I was. Well... Maybe the way in would be to take another look at what I tossed in the trash. Maybe I could try to make some sense of that first. Maybe that's how I—together with you—can gather up the shards of what I really need or want to clarify. If I could just tell you a little bit about what actually happened... Naturally a psychologist in training should have known better. Right? Couldn't I tell what was going on? Couldn't I stop it somehow? You would think I'd have known better... Even though the information I'm about to share is hardly new, if I can keep you with me as I attempt to make sense of what I have to say, then maybe I can begin to put my stupid nightmare down. Do you think?

Trying to Make Sense in Slow Motion

Deep work in a good therapy or analysis is the outcome of surrender and trust emerging in an exclusive intimate environment. Two people are intimately involved in the working through of one person's life. It's no surprise, really, when you come to think about it, that the enterprise itself exposes both partners to a common central question—a natural consequence of such dedicated work. And that question, no matter where it comes from or how embarrassing it feels, is "Why can't we be lovers?"

I believe that every good psychodynamic treatment carries some version of that question, voiced or not, and when we reach it, we know that we have arrived at a critical turning point in the treatment. For the moment at least, we have left the realm of one person pouring out pain, or retreating in the distance, and the other attempting to contain it, of intellectual sparring, tug-of-war head games and heart plays. If treatment continues, a shared enterprise of dedicated work gradually emerges; experiences of intimacy, shared vulnerability, and transference are now *embodied*. We move in and out of embodied states, that is, if we manage to stay together. As we traverse the implicit dangers of new relating, we discover uncharted modes of being, playing, making mistakes, surviving them, and having to strain sometimes to stay awake through heavy hours of boredom. Together we have delineated a particular space between us, an original creation in which we find ourselves able to engage one another in the task at hand, together entering uncharted territory with all its fearful ups and downs.

Of course, mostly for the patient but also for the analyst, the full analytic experience resembles a kind of love story, but you know it's a story with a particular purpose, a story that specifically invites the patient person to revisit those places in childhood where she wanted or never had whatever it was that was lost and whatever might have been that she never mourned; a long-ago place where the self got stuck, stopped growing; a place where vision narrowed just because she didn't know that she had choices about what she wanted or that wanting might not be too much for anybody ... was not bad ...

Ironically, this particular story, evoking interactions that are carefully attended to and whose startling narrative is witnessed by another, requires that as patients we once again give in, go back, relive, surrender to the process precisely in order that we might take authorship of our own present narrative, our own authority in the life we live right now and from here on in. Of course there is a lovesickness that unfolds in this momentous and intimate story. Feelings of love are inherent.

And of course both participants in the process are liable to misconstrue those moments of embodiment, might readily distort the meaning of memory's yearning for lost love. The field is so fragile to begin with and may be so easily trampled.

Yes, I remember, even though it happened many years ago, that as a young intern in my first analysis with a popular and much beloved analyst, I handed my trust over quite immediately, like some innocent kid might hand up for safekeeping her precious toy to the intriguing, scary man. It shames me to think of it. I told my analyst that my open and expressive nature, although gratifying, had led me into unspeakable situations with men—beginning with a parish priest when I was four, and then again with a thirty-three-year-old minister, my camp activities counselor, when I was ten. I told my analyst how much I hated camp, how homesick I felt, but ... I needed to whisper the confession, "I never learned the difference between affection and sexuality." And then (this could have been yesterday ... I remember the words so well), "I think I want to express all my feelings in here without having to worry for once, about its being dangerous to me."

And from behind the couch I heard, "I don't promise not to fuck with you."

"Odd," I thought to myself, I couldn't figure out how to unscramble the double negative in "I don't promise not …" so my mind moved over to focus on "fuck *with* you?" To "fuck you" was one thing—and I could tell that he was not referring to head games—so what did he mean, "to fuck *with* you?" Really odd. I was silent for a while, and then I changed the subject to… I cannot remember.

Some months would pass before the first transgression occurred—a kiss … and then a tongue in my mouth. The next day, I thought I'd make a joke. "Freud would say you had a 'slip of the tongue.'" No response from behind the couch. But at the end of the hour he got up when I got up and did it again! "I don't promise not to fuck with you," I thought to myself as I closed the door behind me (see also B. Pizer, 2000, 2008).

My analyst kept his promise. I mean he broke the thing he said he wouldn't promise. I mean, you get it, don't you? No doubt I felt pretty special at first.

Besides the phenomenon of slow motion, nightmares are probably called so because they happen in the dark. It was very dark in this one, highlighted by the small glow in the distance, like a dusty yellow halo around an old-fashioned streetlamp. I could feel the man come after me, the sound of stalking footsteps, picking up speed as I started to run. I was running for my life when he caught up with me and knocked me flat on the sidewalk where the streetlamp glowed. I screamed as loud as I knew how, but my voice couldn't come out right or make the word *Help*. I kept trying to scream, "Somebody help me!" It seemed to me that now I was able to form the phrase with my mouth, but it came out broken, not loud enough. That truth was horrifying in itself. Where was my voice? I lost my voice! "Help me!" Finally somehow, I escaped his grip before he could do some far worse thing… Running to exhaustion until I dropped. Then blank. Regaining consciousness, I dropped into a hole that became the second part of the nightmare. Or had I fallen into a hold? Another grabbing. I could actually feel the dimensions of the grip, but this time holding from behind—the musculature of strong arms around me. "Help me! Please help me!" Then, from far away, I heard my name, "Barbara." "Help me! Please help. Ohhh … " Sobbing. I felt the arms adjusting to the way I needed them. "Barbara, wake up. You're having a bad dream." "Oh, my God … " Once I realized I could lean back safely in the hold, I heard the sharpness in my crying out, "Where were you?"

"I'm right here," my husband said, "right here." Eyes open now, I couldn't stop trembling... He held me like a baby until finally the trembling went away.

Descriptive and Prescriptive Rules

Here I want to tell you quite directly that I do not believe that as clinicians, teachers, or supervisors, we have been sufficiently schooled in how to deal with and distinguish between love and hate or sexuality and desire in the consulting room, let alone talk freely with colleagues about what happens inside of us as we sit with our patients.

I should say that over the years I have made a particular effort in vivo to fill in for what I perceive as a training gap. In the clinical seminar that I coteach with my husband, I try to flush out the unspeakable as matter-of-factly as I can. "Well, do you love this patient?" I ask. We sense a feeling of relief coming from some of the seminar participants, but from others the question evokes discomfort. Sometimes a supervisee will tell me, blushing, how her patient is unfortunately having "an erotic transference." "Is that like a flu?" I ask lightly—obviously joking. I have the sense that she feels guilty and responsible for having "caused it," having done something wrong. "Do you think it's a sickness?" Another supervisee takes his patient's thinly veiled wish for a kissing relationship in stride. He tells her that he cannot engage in "that way" because it violates the ethics of his profession.

"Do you find her attractive?" I inquire, wishing that such affects could be speakable. "I mean, do you happen to be attracted to her in that way?"

"Yes," he tells me, smiling over his guilt. "It just so happens that I do." Nervous laughter. I remain empathic, focused, wondering. "Could it be she thinks she's doing you a favor by being the one to ask? Or maybe... It's an open question worth our thought, yes?"

He pauses to consider. My supervisee and I are on particularly good terms. We like each other and have worked together for two training years at his request, which makes the boldness of this conversation possible. "Do you think it is unethical," I continue, "for your patient to want you to kiss her? To have that wish?" I work with my supervisee to find his personal comfort and true response to what might well become a turning point in the treatment. He sees that he needs to step forward, not back.

It seems to me that training too often encourages the practice of hiding behind technique and role. To my mind, once you own a feeling and find a word that adequately holds it, you have created a boundary. You have taken a step toward safety in relationship.

My mentor and supervisor, the late Paul Russell, used to make an important distinction between what he called *descriptive* and *prescriptive* rules.

His favorite example: No Smoking on School Premises. (Back in those days, people denied the connection between smoking and health, and cigarettes symbolized manhood or sophistication.) So "No Smoking" in this case is a rule that offers a person only one of two options. You can sneak a cigarette, and if you get caught, you are disobedient or bad; if you do not smoke at school, you are obedient and good. That is to say, obedient and good if you do not smoke or you do but do not get caught. Only two options are available: obedience or disobedience, being good or being bad.

A descriptive rule is different: "If you want to run a marathon, smoking will impact your pace and endurance by X amount." The rest is up to you. This kind of rule becomes a personally guiding framework of relevant information, principles, and probabilities, leaving you with more choices, depending on your relationship to the rule and how it informs your own intentions. By invoking prescriptive and descriptive rules, Russell sought to emphasize our use of rules as an ego function, a competence, rather than a superego function. As he remarked, "The superego is unconscious and, by definition, incompetent" (personal communication). Thus, "I can't engage in sexual activities with you, because it violates the ethics of my profession" gives evidence of a prescriptive rule rather than a clinician's descriptive understanding of his intentions—both personal and professional.

"Why Can't We Be Lovers?"

As far back as 1978, Paul Russell—a graduate of the Boston Psychoanalytic Institute who taught the Freud course to first-year candidates—delivered his paper "The Negotiation of Affect" (Russell, 1978/2006). In it, he claimed that "negotiation" superseded the older notions of a one-person analytic interpretation. An extensive quote is relevant here.

> Every treatment delivers with varying poignancy and intensity, its own particular version of the question "Why can't we be lovers?" It is a painful question that is defended against by both patient and therapist. It is a real question, not simply a transferential one, and must be negotiated, not simply analyzed [or denied, I would add]. (p. 626)

Russell continued, "Therapist and patient cannot be lovers for reasons that are very close to the reason parent and child cannot be lovers. It must be accepted and mourned in order for other, possible love relationships to occur" (p. 626). Here is where the process of relating supersedes specific content. Russell went on to say,

> The patient, to begin with, may not be able to *feel* this. Like a parent, the therapist may be the only one who is able to feel it. But the child *needs* [emphasis added] the parent to feel it with enough containing consistency to create a situation where the child will eventually feel it in him or herself, *not as some kind of rule* [emphasis added] but simply as what follows from an even deeper wish, namely to continue to grow. To think of it as a rule, loses the quieter, more powerful organizing negotiation that is inherent. Negotiation is a clarifying, individuating process. The fact that negotiation is happening, let alone the results of negotiation, are all *new structure* that is growth and development. (p. 626)

And as Russell (1996) emphasized elsewhere, "Structure is the passage of process with involvement" (p. 216).

But here in this early paper (1978/2006), Russell spoke with equal fervor about affects—the centrality of affect in human relatedness. Yes, we are born with feelings, but we must be taught to *own* them, rather than project them into others—pawning them off. If we cannot own our feelings, we are liable to enact them. How, in our growing up, have we learned to own and respect what we feel? And if these lessons were not taught throughout our development, how are we taught/trained to use what we feel in the work we do? How do we, as therapists and analysts, own our feelings in such a way that we can use them creatively? Are we permitted to love our patients without such love turning over into making love concretely or, in the vernacular, having sex? Surely, however we answer, as clinicians we need to ask ourselves the question. We need to create an environment in which the issue of love and loving can be safely explored.

Process with Involvement

I know that my second analysis provided much repair to the damage I had suffered in the first. And yet, I have to say, something I would have wished for was missing. I believe that my second analyst felt like he had to hold back from me.

Together we realized that a part of my experience was due to a deeply familiar transference. Growing up, my mother held back. I can still catch the scent of her soap, the softness of her skin as I snuggled up against her while she stroked my hair for what seemed like a small forever. And for a long time I thought I understood what my father meant when he would see us like that and make the musing comment, "Barbara, can't you ever have enough? Can't you ever have enough?" I accepted his premise (a question always posed in the negative) as my deficiency until many years later when I sat with mother—still beautiful in her eighties—in a hospital waiting room. She came to Boston to be tested for Alzheimer's. As we sat there waiting, she turned to me and—out of the blue— remarked, "Barbara, did I ever tell you that I was sexually abused by my older brother from age five to eight?" "What?" I gasped, despite long season- ing as a psychologist. "Have you told Daddy this?" "Yes," she replied, "last week."

So, in her growing dementia, my mother gave me a great gift. She let me know why she couldn't bear expressions of affection, especially physical ones. She let me know that braiding my hair was never a problem, but my endless requests for stroking caused her to recoil inside. I could see now that it was not the *quantity* of time I needed in her lap, it was the *quality* of her stroking that kept me there, waiting for what was not to come.

Do you suppose that if, by some outlandish miracle, my mother had told me (or at least told herself!) her story when I was four years old, I would have been spared the trauma bestowed on me by her and the parish priest? Do you think my mother's story contributed to why I introduced myself to each of my training supervisors as a survivor of sexual abuse? A priest, a minister, an analyst, and indirectly my mother's brother.

Even though I believe we all carry the *potential* for boundary crossings or boundary violations, some of us are less immune than others, and as I began this work, I had reason to engage my supervisors' help in keeping an eye on my interactions with patients.

As for my second analyst, transference notwithstanding, I actually think, because of the first aborted treatment, he was afraid to give expression to his feelings during our work. My second analysis was truly a good one, but I cannot deny that something was missing. Was my second analyst afraid to love me? Mostly in the early sessions I felt clumsy, like a person who could not be loved, was not lovable, soiled by my first analysis. We would have to move through this dilemma in some way, and ultimately we did.

We reached our own version of that turning point I spoke of earlier, an embodiment that I took in. (I reserve elaboration of that story for another time. See Chapter 9.)

Love and Do No Harm

Today, as an analyst, I experience a strange and consistent phenomenon among the number of trauma patients I have treated. Comparatively speaking, my *n* is small, which is why I ask you to consider whether I'm completely off base. Among my trauma patients, I have found that they move around the world with an air of what I can only call "innocence." A kind of wide-eyed aura that seems to coexist dissociatively with hypervigilance, startle, and, often, flat affect. The people I'm referring to have suffered and survived. They are not martyrs. They have an open, trusting way about them that seems to remain unshaken, a fresh readiness to risk if it makes sense, a curiosity and unselfconscious courage, and they show surprise when I point it out. One can easily explain the trouble they are liable to get into as a "repetition compulsion," or a defensive maneuver, but even so I want to insist that there's more to it—this air of innocence. Maybe this group of patients, like myself, shares a similar legacy, that is, the transgenerational transmission of trauma, an alien identification (Faimberg, 2005) that surely contributes to their air of innocence. I do not know. But could there be some neurobiological basis, do you suppose, a predisposition expressed in this way? What do you suppose?

On January 26, 2012, *Commonwealth Magazine* posted an online newsflash in boldface letters: "Sex with patient caused no harm, doctor says" (Herman, 2012). This doctor, "a heavyweight in the world of psychiatry," met with his patient up to six times a week in analysis and told her that "she was the most important person in his life " He insisted, "He did her and her husband no harm." When the patient argued that "she lacked the ability to recognize that she was being harmed as a result of … transference," the doctor was "flabbergasted." "Unbelievable!" he said, continuing,

> Dr. X was not mentally ill … has been a licensed psychologist for two years before the alleged affair took place… [She,] a professional who has been trained in handling the transference phenomenon, cannot seriously claim that she was not … fully cognizant of what happened during her training analysis.

The Nightmare Is Such a Shame

"Really?" I want to say, with the familiar inflection I'm getting used to hearing from my patients these days. "Really?"

All right. Now I feel freer to tell you my nightmare's crazy dialogue—that came clear only on the following afternoon. Do you know what that bad guy says to me when he gets me down by the lamppost? (Good thing I do not have to look at you when I tell.) This man, dead serious and with evil intent and threatening tone, says to me, he says to me, "Okay, I'm going to pee all over you!"

The second part of the nightmare gets worse, sillier and more horrifying. This is the part that happens when my husband has put his arms around me—back to front—but I go on in the nightmare a little longer. I haven't escaped the monster who is after me. His echo-y voice reverberates.

"And now"—just picture this guy, his face in my face, above me, and suddenly, with no warning, his face is gone to where I can only feel it right behind me, nose in my hair, words in my ear. What's he going to do to me? Now he tells me, and I start to shake—"Now I am going to burp in your ear!"

That's it! Now that I think of it, I have to laugh, because laughing is the only way I can shake it off.

I'm so embarrassed, and I'm laughing! This very minute I associate to as long ago as I can remember. Sometime soon after toilet training, I imagine. I can still see myself in the garden playing. I have a yellow ruffled sunsuit on. Happily playing in the fantasyland of fairies and flowers and trees. I feel the feel of increasing pressure happening around my bottom. I do not want to go inside. Do not want to. The garden is sunny; inside the house feels dark. There is a big evergreen tree I could hide behind. I do not know how high it is, but the tip of the top seems to touch the sun, and its branches are full and wide. If I just get myself behind that green bunker, I can pull off my ruffles and squat down with nobody the wiser. Yes.

But I forgot to think about the window on the second floor of the house. I was squatting when I heard the tap-tap-tap from that window above my head. The sharp metallic clicking of my mother's wedding ring as she tap-tap-tapped my S.O.S. against the glass. She caught me in trouble. I do not remember what happened after that. But I can still feel the sting of shame in my cheeks.

I have another association to the nightmare and its ridiculous threat of burping in my ear. (By the way, I suspect that the word *burp* is a dream-work product, a kind of age-appropriate cleanup of the more descriptive term *belch*.) I am in second grade at school. Joyce Polanski sits behind me in the third row.

One morning, at my desk, I feel a slender geyser of warm liquid shoot into my ear. Like lightning strikes before you hear the thunder, I know exactly what is happening before I hear the retching sound of Joyce Polanski throwing up. Warm spurts in my ear. I couldn't turn around. That's when Mrs. Osman says right in front of the whole class that I am an example of thoughtlessness. I didn't turn around to help my poor neighbor who was being sick. I just sit there, shuddering, hands over my ears, elbows on my knees, and knees shaking all over the place. I am unable to say a word to Mrs. Osman, who makes it clear I should be ashamed of myself, and I am. I cannot speak to say to her what happened. I'm breathing through my mouth, and there is goo inside my left hand. I do not know what to do. Paralyzed, I wince when I feel Joyce leaning forward toward me once again. I can still hear her as she whispers as close to my ear as she can get, "I forgot to brush my teeth," by way of an apology.

When the Price of Love Becomes a Loss of Love

It does seem to me that traumas and nightmares move in slow motion. We get that sense because in both instances there is too much to process all at once, so all we can do is slow things down or cover our ears. I do not think about "slippery slopes"; that is not where my mind wants to go. I am more inclined to think about training our affects, wording them, owning them rather than passing them over, choosing how and what to say when we can. I think about descriptive rules that bring real life into the prescription of a necessary ethics code.

In my experience ($n = 1$), sexual boundary violations in a clinical context violently penetrate the delicate intrapsychic membrane between adulthood and the person who once long ago was a small child seeking nurture and love. And I believe that the thing of value first sought after, the first thing that feels to me closest to the word *love*, is more like *encirclement*, literally *like arms around your newborn self that create your first experience of boundaries— boundaries that contain and connect*. The clinical context, Winnicott's (1965) holding environment, it seems to me, begins with this maternal metaphor. And do you agree from your experience that whenever you trade encirclement—given or received—for whatever else masquerades as love, you'll pay a price for it? The basic need for love gets lost, and that price turns out to be too high.

So I began this article by asking you what might be useful to convey from my experience, and now the narrative appears more helpful *to me* than I first anticipated. But maybe you too can take to heart my sense that you just do not "get over" traumas. Rather, you try to metabolize them over and over, and each time they return, you get a brief jolt to stop and question some more. Where and how do you carry the perpetrator within yourself? What part do you play in calling trauma back? It seems as if there is always more to master, such as slowly letting go of shame, turning triggers into signals that something is amiss within or without. I keep coming up with new questions to think about and grow on. My nightmare, for example, occurred as a result of this writing assignment, starkly presenting me with new elements to process.

Although all nightmares may share common themes of terror, shame, and helplessness, I detect another dimension in the structure of my nightmare, as evidenced through the dual structure of my memory system. On waking, the dream images were clear, unrepressed. I associated directly to my first analyst's assault, complete with tremors. But I didn't realize then how the dream dialogue remained unformulated, dormant in memory's other channel. Trauma memory. Both in real time and in the intrapsychic passage of time, the dream dialogue came out of dissociation only on the following afternoon—perhaps triggered by the sound of innocent children, home from school, yelping.

My peculiar nightmare's unboundaried penetration into the deep past illustrates a kind of unconsciously driven "living proof" of separate memory systems and brings to mind my tentative notion of a relationship between traumatic experiences and a particular air of innocence, as well as furthering thoughts about what I call "encirclement."

I have reviewed Paul Russell's ideas about descriptive and prescriptive rules as a way to emphasize that reliance on our ethics code is necessary but not sufficient for educating new clinicians or safeguarding limits for senior analysts who consider themselves above the law, entitled, and exceptional enough to make their own rules as they go along. When I confessed to my first analyst that I didn't know the difference between affection and sexuality, I was not aware that he didn't either. What we need across the board is more training and more checks and balances around the depth and density of affects—how to distinguish and express them in ways that will help our patients grow and thrive. In other words, how might we be trained to use ourselves creatively within the conventions and constraints of our profession? How and when is love speakable in a clinical context? What role does the transgenerational transmission of trauma play in the way we handle clinical difficulties? Are the therapist's sexual feelings abnormal? How might they be healthily processed? How much do we share with our patients? How do we distinguish between limits and inhibitions? These are just a few of the questions for us to review and revisit again and again, for life.

But the time has come for me to rest my case for now. I will do so by quoting my final emphatic statement, spoken directly to my abuser at the Board of Registration in Medicine on September 9, 1992.

When I read Respondent's Memorandum Regarding Sanctions, I was once again distressed and offended to encounter Dr. X's unrelenting rationale for his sexual behavior with me. Dr. X continues to insist that his is a special case in which love between himself, as analyst, and me, his patient, justifies seduction and intercourse.

According to Dr. X's lawyer, "substantial evidence of record" supports his construction of a "true love" theory of defense. Attorney Y quotes from the record his client's statement that "I loved her passionately." Then my cross-examination is quoted in some detail as a way of substantiating this notion of an exceptional situation that places it outside of ordinary codes of ethics or law. After establishing that Dr. X hugged me in the first six months of treatment, that I felt loved by him and was thrilled by it, and I quote: "You found, as you expressed, comfort and solace from your relationship, with Dr. X. That is so, isn't it?" I said then, as I say now, "Yes it is."

I would like to say to this Board that just as Dr. X stated elsewhere in his testimony that the love between us was obvious to others, the love between Dr. X and his adolescing daughter, which I witnessed over the years, was also obvious to others and to me. Given the nature of their relationship, this was entirely appropriate. But had he taken advantage of her frank adoration of him and dependence upon him, he would have caused—as with me—irreparable damage that would haunt her throughout her life and her relationships. I believe he would not take such advantage of his daughter's vulnerable feelings.

He did take advantage of mine.

Still at this late date, Dr. X seems not to comprehend the destructiveness of his behavior toward me, and his profession, in the name of love. His rationale for a sexual relationship with me, his patient, is a perversion of love; furthermore, it constitutes a destructive insult to the invaluable healing power of love and respect in the therapeutic relationship.

The final statement in Memorandum Regarding Sanctions concludes: "In the interest of justice, Dr. X requests this Board to refrain from revoking and/or suspending his license to practice medicine." Now, it is neither my business nor my intention to speak here today regarding the particular form of discipline to be taken in this case. But I simply *cannot* allow to go unchallenged the implication that Dr. X's "passionate love" for me and my natural dependent love for him provide any moral or ethical justification for his violation of me. I can no longer take any pride in the love I once felt for him; and I feel *further* devalued and degraded by his insistence that love was the currency of exchange in the shameful occurrences between us.

Dr. X lost his license, as did many others like him, though they continue to practice without it. I have spoken my piece (peace?), and that in itself is a relief. In telling my nightmare, I have put it to rest. Put it to rest until the next time. I find that good enough.

References

Faimberg, H. (2005). *The telescoping of generations*. London/New York, NY: Routledge.

Herman, C. M. (2012, January 26). Sex with patient caused no harm, doctor says. *Commonwealth Magazine*.

Pizer, B. (2000). The therapist's routine consultations: A necessary window in the treatment frame. *Psychoanalytic Dialogues, 10*, 197–207. http://dx.doi.org/10.1080/10481881009348531

Pizer, B. (2008). The heart of the matter in matters of the heart: Power and intimacy in analytic and couple relationships. *International Journal of Psychoanalytic Self Psychology, 3*, 304–319. http://dx.doi.org/10.1080/ 15551020802108653

Russell, P. L. (1996). Process with involvement: The interpretation of affect. In L. Lifson (Ed.), *Understanding therapeutic action: Psychodynamic concepts of cure* (pp. 201–216). Hillsdale, NJ: The Analytic Press.

Russell, P. L. (2006). The negotiation of affect. *Contemporary Psychoanalysis, 42*, 621–636. (Delivered as unpublished paper in 1978)

Winnicott, D. W. (1965). *The maturational processes and the facilitating environment*. New York, NY: International Universities Press.

Reverie

Who Would Think

Who would think how useless, how unbelievable, one's reaching out could become? I know it's not that loving is the problem. I know you know the way to love. The trouble is the state you get in when you need the most is just exactly where you've been consistently unmet, and so of course the safest place to be is all alone.

I guess the thing I have to learn again and again is not to search for "ways to make it better." It's hard to put away desire while remaining present. Not to feel somehow unwieldy, *not to act*, to hold in mind the exhortation to Bo Peep—"leave them alone and they'll come home"—and keep believing that with quiet constancy and caring the prediction might come true.

DOI: 10.4324/9781032666303-22

Not-Me

The Vicissitudes of Aging[1]

Introduction

The experience of Old Age, once you have reached that time of life, does not creep up on you; it's already there in your body before you stop to notice. It's up to you when you decide to notice how you wear your aging process, how you own it and, if you do, whether you dare experience the emotions that come along with growing old.

I want to tell you about a few ways you might find yourself more able to admit your years, take in what you've lost, what you've left behind, or what you've been left with holding all alone. I want to suggest a few tools that you could use to help accommodate this later life state of aging with a modicum of grace. And I want to warn you about the very real danger that you and I and, eventually, each and every one of us is liable to fall prey to.

Of course I realize that the tasks we face in coming to grips with the vicissitudes of aging are far too complex to address all at once in this small space and time. And yet we have the opportunity to think together for a moment, to associate from observation or experience, to try and make some sense of what it means to grow up full of dreams only to grow old; to share an idea or two, and maybe even develop a few tentative hypotheses to offer up for questioning. And, for the sake of enlightenment, we might even begin to speak the unspeakable surrounding the vicissitudes of aging.

Here Is One Association

I must have been somewhere in my late fifties, or maybe middle sixties, when a fairly recent colleague stopped by to spend a day with us before going on to New York. Why she and I were standing in the bedroom I have no idea but this colleague caught sight of a photograph on my husband, Stuart's, dresser. I watched her as she moved in to take a closer look.

DOI: 10.4324/9781032666303-23

"Wow," she exclaimed, astonished. "Who is *that*?"

"Well, it's on his dresser," I replied coyly. "Who do you think it is?"

"I don't know." For a split second, my colleague feigned a frogmouth, "She's so beautiful," and then her lips turned over into a playful grin. "C'mon, who *is* she?"

"It's me," I said, embarrassed and proud at the same time.

"That was YOU?" *she cried, astonished.* **"I can't believe it!"**

Blushing is rare for me but I could feel the blood rising up in my cheeks. What did she mean by *"was"*? Could she not connect my older self to the person in the picture? An anxious pause between us. What became of who I was? What in the world had I turned into? I felt angry, I felt bad, hurt... Now I remember that my colleague was smiling. I believe she thought she had paid me a great compliment.

A Childhood Memory and the Facts of Life

Paradoxically perhaps, our sense-making efforts hardly ever emerge in a straight line. Life and growth are more circuitous than that, more chaotic and mysterious. I remember as a ten-year-old (having never heard of photomicrography) believing, hoping, that if I sat quietly and long enough in front of a springtime bud, I'd be able to witness its gradual opening into petals, and then, after the requisite days of blooming without me, I'd come back to my post and train my focus on the flower's gradual droop or giving up of tension just before its petals fell. For more reasons than the obvious, no matter how hard or repeatedly I tried, I never could succeed in these botanical experiments and—truth be told—despite how much I wished it were otherwise, a big part of me *expected* to fail. My grade-school teachers always told me I was a mediocre student with no patience for the sciences. No bones about it, I was a bad student so that was that.

I believe these two stories begin to suggest the pitfalls inherent in the aging process, or to put it bluntly, our last chances to risk new understandings about ourselves. But before we take a theoretical leap into a description of vicissitudes, let me provide one more metaphor for the trouble we are liable to get into. You know the one. You're walking along an elegant city street on a bright afternoon when a figure in a display window catches your eye. Just like my recent colleague, you move in closer to have a look. The sun has arranged itself in such a way that what you see in the window is the figure and face of yourself looking back at you and you are shocked. Face to face, you are forced to recognize the discrepancy between this scraggly stranger in the window and whom you know yourself to be inside.

And by the way, to whisper the unspeakable, right after the shop-window shock, you might go home to check it out, only to discover that one's mirror is less cloudy and more merciless. See how the outer body shrinks and crinkles. There's the thinning out of hair and, the fullness of passion notwithstanding, the most vulnerable precious place at your age is reminiscent of a prepubescent child.

A Theoretical Scaffold and the Work of Harry Stack Sullivan

Sociologist/philosopher George Herbert Mead (1863–1931) hypothesized—in contrast to biologically based views of his contemporaries—a social theory of the self as emerging out of social interactions. Inspired by Mead, Harry Stack Sullivan (1892–1949) built his interpersonal theory. Sullivan (1953) declared that the self is comprised of the reflected appraisals of others. Therefore, the evolution of a person's self-regard is a social phenomenon that gets communicated from the outside and translated on the inside by parts of self (today we might call them self-states) that Sullivan referred to as "Personifications." Personifications are formed by our responses to the reactions we receive from our environment that we split into shapes of "good-me," "bad-me," and—when faced with unspeakable anxiety—"not-me."[2]

Briefly stated and oversimplified (see Sullivan, 1953), the infant who is loved and responded to on the basis of expressed need, such as "crying-when-hungry," experiences the tenderness of the "mothering one." Cumulatively, the infant's experience of such positive regard, valuing, and nourishment forms an emergent "personification" of good-me. The good-me is sustained and developed through the growing child's experiences of being valued. The bad-me comes on line as the growing child engages in activities that evoke parental anxiety over risks or violations of social norms or expectations. Good-me and bad-me join to form what Sullivan calls the self-system, a dynamism designed to shape experience to minimize anxiety. So it is the bad-me personification in the self-system that the child learns to avoid. And the greater the anxiety induced in the parent, the greater the child's incentive to navigate away from the deepest waters of bad-me.

However, it is all too common that parents, traumatized and unresolved by their translation of social norms, may react to certain behaviors, states, or affects in their child with such a high degree of overwhelming anxiety that the child is exposed to unbearable, "uncanny" distress. The self that is induced by these extremely anxious states in the parent cannot be tolerated by the child and, therefore, cannot be experienced as a part of me. Sullivan (1953) refers to this phantom personification, held apart in the realm of dissociation, as the not-me.[3]

But I want to point out that even as personifications play their part in shaping curtailment of accessible experience, Sullivan's theory includes a distinct hopefulness that subsequent unfolding experience in the course of development—development divided and defined by seven developmental stages, each of which provides the opportunity for personality change—may modify the personification bad-me.

Nevertheless, we must remember that the sealed off self-state not-me lies hidden until further notice, endangering growth or change. Sullivan's not-me corresponds to our contemporary conception of dissociation or dis-identification. "This is *not* who I am!"

What I hope to show you is how a particular not-me dissociative process that is likely to occur specifically in relation to growing old is anathema to living. Any approach that might permit the mind to drop down (or across!) into not-me generates an intolerable anxiety that mobilizes urgent exclusion from self-experience. The not-me belongs to someone else who sits in a black hole and threatens to suck us in, sucks us dry of all vitality. Consider this description by Donnel B. Stern (2010):

> the person one must not be—the self-state one must not find oneself inhabiting—is someone who felt disappointed, bereft, frightened, humiliated, shamed, or otherwise threatened. *One must not be the person to whom that thing happened, the person who has feelings, memories, and experience that comes with being that person.* (p. 13, emphasis added)

So it is the personification not-me that bars experience, subverting new growth as we age toward our final opportunities in living life. As we get older and supposedly wiser, we become in fact more vulnerable to the seduction of not-me, and as long as experience remains in dissociation, the reflectiveness that might lead to acceptance or change goes missing.

Regarding Sullivan's (1953) self-system, here is a critical quote to hold in mind:

> When I talk about the self-system, I want it clearly understood that I am talking about a *dynamism* which comes to be enormously important in understanding interpersonal relations. This dynamism is an explanatory conception: it is not a thing, a region, or what not, such as superegos egos, ids and so on. Among the things this conception explains is something that can't be described as a quasientity, the personification of the self. The personification of the self is what you are talking about when you talk about yourself as "I," and what you are often, if not invariably, referring to when you talk about "me" and "my." But I would like to make it forever clear that the relation of personifications to that which is personified is always complex and sometimes multiple, and that personifications are not adequate descriptions of that which is personified! (p. 167)

The "Old-Me"

So, in the spirit of Sullivan's conceptual model, let us entertain the idea of a fourth personification that sits right next to not-me because it does not make an appearance until life's last developmental epoch. As a way of softening the inevitable, I playfully name this personification "old-me"![4] (But I couldn't be more serious.) Like all other personifications of self, old-me derives from the reflected appraisals of others. It stands to reason then that the old-me is formed by an aging person's experience of anxiety emanating from the environment or a particular important other, as the other's representation of us is destabilized by the physical changes that they see. Perhaps a *memento mori*. We move more slowly, which means it's harder to catch up. It takes us more time to remember where we put things. To some extent, the anxiety induced in the other by our manifestations of aging may exist along a gradient of bad-me severity. But I think we have to face the unfortunate fact that signs of aging in us all too often evoke an uncanny anxiety in *others*. And, thereby, *as our experience of self continues to be shaped by the reflected appraisals of others, uncanny levels of anxiety in others coerce an entire area of dissociation in our self-experience.*

In this day and age, there are, of course, a myriad of ways to cover up— creams and wigs, surgeries and youthful clothes. Nothing wrong with any of this as long as we can remember who we are inside. The important thing is to manage not to disown old-me, or surreptitiously slide the experience of our aging into the realm of not-me. Whenever we begin to approach the experience of our dissociated old-me, we need to recognize our suffering of uncanny emotions with some compassion as we endure the shame, the dread, the loathing and disgust—the reflected appraisal of others conveyed through the medium of barely tolerable anxiety.

Some Tools for Maintaining an Aging Self ("Good Old-Me")

Here is my action plan, my tool kit for mindful aging:

1. Creative Planning for the Future
   (Tomorrow, next week, six months, next year)
2. Making Space for Memory, Grief, and Transformation
3. Learning to Accept Help with Grace
4. Negotiating Balance Between Denial and Acceptance

I illustrate in a final vignette.

Climbing Gorham Mountain

In Bar Harbor, Maine, where we go for a month in the summer, the evenings stay clear and bright past eight o'clock. Over the years, at dinner during the last week of our stay, we ask the ritual question: What was our favorite experience of the vacation and what was our biggest regret? This last summer Stuart told me that his biggest regret was loss of our climb up Gorham Mountain. Why? I asked … we still have five days left.

I knew full well why and didn't want to say. Stuart had already told me that his trick knee, from a fall on black ice two years ago, had gotten worse. Unpredictably, it could collapse with jabbing pain while climbing. Now at the table in Bar Harbor, we were both quiet. And in the pause I suddenly flashed on our first climb some forty years ago. Mount Cardigan (in New Hampshire. Actually, it was Stuart's first climb. City boy meets country girl. Or rather, years of summer camp, of hiking and climbing and swimming. I trusted my body in the same way that Stuart trusted his mind. He was the one who taught me that I was not too dumb to apply to graduate school, and I was the one who helped him overcome his fear of heights.

Mount Cardigan. Just now, approaching the first stand of evergreens, we can feel the light dust of a new snow as it brushes across our cheeks. Stuart begins to laugh. "Holy shit!" A curse of surprise and delight uniquely his own. "What?" I say. "The trees," he says. "The only time I saw a bunch of trees all crowded together like that was as a kid in Rego Park on an empty lot where they were selling Christmas trees!"

Now, as I looked at him sitting at the table across from me, I was flooded with images of our mountain hiking over the years and the gradual reversal of who helped whom over the rocks and along the trails. "It gives me such pleasure," Stuart said, "to get the chance to repay you. For *me* to be the one to help *you* in the rocky places. *How cool is that?*"

"Pretty cool," I thought.

"I could go up myself," Stuart broke into my reverie, "and somehow manage my knee. But I can't trust myself to be stable support to help you." A pause. And then, "suppose my trick knee buckles just when I'm supporting you?"

"We'd be Jack and Jill," I said, wistfully.

My mother was a mountain climber. She did the Alps ... she taught me all the tricks she knew. Like not to sit down when you tire on the trail. Stand sideways on the incline, have a few raisins. . .

Stuart paid the check and we walked along Main Street to purchase an evening latte.

I took a deep breath and told him, "You go in, okay?"

Another breath and, "I'll wait out here."

He went inside Choco-latte.

I had noticed that nextdoor Cadillac Hiking Guides was still open. With trepidation, I moved toward the door of Cadillac Hiking Guides.

I should tell you that whenever I feel embarrassed, I tend to raise my voice. I don't know why. Maybe it's to drown out what I don't want to hear myself saying. Or maybe to keep myself afloat so I don't fall through the floor in shame. I opened the door to Cadillac Hiking Guides and stood by it, stock still. The desk was about twenty feet away at the opposite wall. I took another deep breath and then,

"Is there anybody around here would be prepared to help an eighty-year-old lady up a mountain?" I shouted.

There was.
"Sure."

I held my two tickets for Saturday morning like one would hold a hand of cards.

Stuart was just coming out to the sidewalk with our lattes when I approached him with the two tickets and a plan.

"And you can't get out of it," I said, "I've already paid."

"*Holy shit*," he told me, grinning.

Postscript

I close with Mary Oliver's "The Summer Day" from *House of Light* (1992):

Who made the world?
Who made the swan, and the black bear?
Who made the grasshopper?
This grasshopper, I mean—
the one who has flung herself out of the grass,
the one who is eating sugar out of my hand,
who is moving her jaws back and forth instead of up and down—
who is gazing around with her enormous and complicated eyes.
Now she lifts her pale forearms and thoroughly washes her face.
Now she snaps her wings open, and floats away.
I don't know exactly what a prayer is.
I do know how to pay attention, how to fall down
into the grass, how to kneel in the grass,
how to be idle and blessed, how to stroll through the fields,
which is what I have been doing all day.
Tell me, what else should I have done?
Doesn't everything die at last, and too soon?
Tell me, what is it you plan to do
with your one wild and precious life?

(p. 60)

Notes

1 An earlier version of this chapter was presented at a Plenary Panel on "Aging and Its Vicissitudes," Annual Conference, The International Association for Relational Psychoanalysis and Psychotherapy, Sydney, Australia, May 28, 2017.

2 In *Blind Spot* (Banaji & Greenwald, 2016), a report of current research on hidden biases—race, gender, age, etc.,—the researchers conclude, "A preference for the young among the elderly is further evidence that the outside ends up inside the mind" (p. 68).
3 Given my particular emphasis that authentic communication—both verbal and nonverbal—originates in an experience that I call "Body Words"(Chapter 15), I quote what Sullivan (1953 has to say about Personifications: "Now here I have set up three aspects of interpersonal cooperation which are necessary for the infant's survival, and which dictate learning. Infants are customarily exposed to all of these before the era of infancy is finished. From experience of these three sorts —with rewards, with the anxiety gradient, and with practically obliterative sudden severe anxiety—there comes an initial personification of three phases of what presently will be *me*, that which is invariably connected with the sentience of *my body*—and you will remember that *my body* as an organization of experience has come to be distinguished from everything else by its self-sentient character.... Now at this time, the beginning Personifications of *me* are good-me, bad-me, and not-me.... [I]n this or another culture, it is rather inevitable that there shall be this tripartite cleavage in Personifications, which have as their central tie—the thing that binds them ultimately into one, that always keeps them in very close relation—their relatedness to the growing conception of 'my body'" (p. 161).
4 Perhaps by rights we should think of "old-me" only as a developmental epoch rather than fooling around with an added personification. My intention here is not to build out Sullivan's theory by adding a missing personification; rather, I am using Sullivan's model metaphorically to describe a self-state in which we identify our self as old-me. Our experience of old seems to have become more flexible than one's actual years and more dependent on self and other perception. Note that Freud considered anyone over forty as middle aged while these days retirement age is no longer bound to sixty-five. I note as well that while in this developmental epoch, physical "renovations" become more possible, wisdom may allow us to broaden or alter our perceptions of self and other!

References

Banaji, M. R., & Greenwald, A. G. (2016). *Blindspot: Hidden biases of good people*. New York, NY: Bantam Books.
Oliver, M. (1992). *House of light: Poems by Mary Oliver*. Boston, MA: Beacon Press.
Stern, D. B. (2010). *Partners in thought*. New York, NY: Routledge.
Sullivan, H. S. (1953). *The interpersonal theory of psychiatry*. New York, NY: W.W. Norton & Co.

Reverie

Whatever the Rewards of Childhood

Whatever the rewards of childhood—and for some of us there may be many—we have to understand that growing up is also more or less a form of torture. Especially when you dare to undertake the enterprise of becoming your own person.

"Learning your lesson" is the mommy and the daddy of untold mistakes. And the second or third time you make the same mistake, even if by accident, you know you need to be ashamed of yourself.

Will somebody please tell me how to be your own person and play it safe at the same time? In whose eyes are you "good," and who will tell you if you've got it "right"?

Whatever you do, however you feel—if that is still an option—keep in mind the old familiar rhyme you heard in grade school.

I'm rubber, you're glue.
Whatever you say
Jumps off of me
And sticks to you.

Of course, it never really works, but it's a first-line defense that gives you a small reprieve, a moment, at least, to get your bearings.

DOI: 10.4324/9781032666303-24

Body Words

Transforming the Unspeakable in Clinical Process

There is a reason I want to tell you about what happened with my patient Doreen and me. I almost let myself lose her sooner than I actually did, and I really think I would have lost her earlier had I not been writing about what we were trying to accomplish in a once-a-week treatment situation.

I also need to tell you about a repetitious fantasy, a little secret that I carried with me in my first years as a clinician. Sitting with a patient in my consulting room, I fantasized an ideal supervisor, or maybe a whole group of supervisors, behind a one-way mirror watching over me. I would feel so much safer in their gaze, free to listen and engage as I do with an embodied felt sense of the moment, the process, and the immediacy of my experience (Gendlin, 1964). I could bring this felt immediacy to whatever it was that I found within me and risked to say to my patient, because the experts observing behind the mirror would take note. The experts would mark down and hold in mind what I said, how it flowed (or didn't), and how the patterns and directions of our process assumed shape and meaning. From their more aerial view of our process close-up on the ground, they would be able to guide and supervise thoughtfully what I was doing in the moment.

I don't know exactly when it dawned on me that my note taking after sessions and journaling in the blue book I keep above my desk provide much of what I was in fantasy hoping to gain. For me, the act of translating what happens in the consulting room into a language that comes as close as possible to living experience is no small task, and I use that process to supervise myself. Knowing that I will be writing later, knowing I'll be taking the position behind the one-way mirror observing myself gives me the freedom to be fully present and spontaneous in the field with my patient.

At right around the time Doreen and I began to see each other, I found myself rooting around in my blue journal, seeking to find a shorthand

DOI: 10.4324/9781032666303-25

expression for the astonishing thing that happens in the light of genuine experiencing. I mean when analyst or patient suddenly breaks through an ancient and repetitious way of responding and comes up with a word or phrase or sentence that unlocks a stuck place, that opens up a vista of experiencing that neither partner in the dyad had anticipated. The metaphor that I came up with, the name that I find useful is *Body Words*.

Body Words gather up the fragments of what may be only vaguely felt at first, emerging into a word, gesture, or phrase that suddenly appears from nowhere, "unbidden" (Stern, 1997). Body Words signal a transformative experience heading toward increased integration of inner and outer processes, of direct experience and representation. Let me reiterate that what I call Body Words is an experience I think of as having the shape of an arc. I use Body Words to indicate the peak of an experience that travels from inside to outside.

Developmentally, Body Words evolve from the first conversations held within each one of us as we attempt to make meaning of the world as it enters through our senses from the outside and as we answer to it with feelings from the inside. It is a conversation that develops naturally enough until or unless something intercepts like trauma or exposure to shame; or maybe an early pattern of misrecognition begins to skew the internal dialogue, or subtle punishments inhibit. Any and all of these strictures have an impact on the words or gestures that we make or experience, gradually, imperceptibly, cutting us loose from what once was truly felt, encouraging forgetfulness of how or what we meant to say—if anything at all. The end result becomes a disembodied language either so shocking or by now so ordinary that we dissociatively disattend the unhooked dialogue in others and ourselves until or unless we are lucky enough to stumble on a particular moment when we are jolted awake or aware.

I hope to illustrate the meaning and function of Body Words through my own narrative of scenes from a treatment. It is my story, and I don't know what Doreen might say about it, because some time after giving me permission to write about us, her husband was transferred to another city, and she and her family moved away.

Body Words and the Treatment Process

Maybe I'm afraid to dive right into the initial interactions between Doreen and me. I did feel inadequate for quite a while and yes, a well of shame, but there is more to be said about Body Words, a natural source of vitality that in our growing up can often atrophy and register in our consulting rooms as a peculiar unease. My mentor Paul Russell tells us that we are born with feelings, but we have to learn to own them—or not. And here I am talking about a way that we communicate the details of our feelings that may or may not reflect Body Words.

As I have already indicated, Body Words suggest an innate integration of body and mind. Authentic meaning in the present takes the form of Body Words. The presence or absence of Body Words within the self and in conversation with others is clearly felt and yet remains elusive, which is peculiar, since the concept simply expresses an energetic sense of feeling real in the moment. We know the moment when we feel it—we feel "in touch." Our contact with ourself or another has a genuine ring to it. And we don't necessarily know the minute when we don't feel real or present with our self or another, or we discover our absence too late. That is, Body Words evolve in inverse proportion to the repetition compulsion.

Russell (2006a) emphasizes that "the concept of the repetition compulsion is so basic, and yet so far reaching that it cuts across every level of any given theory" (p. 604). Furthermore,

> one could say that every theoretical addition, contribution, perspective, if it's worth its salt, will have to say something about the nature, the structure, the etiology of the repetition compulsion. The concept of the repetition compulsion I take to be the most important concept Freud left to us. (p. 604)

I suggest there is a dialectic between what I call Body Words and the Repetition Compulsion, a dialectic that becomes one of the primary organizers of every transformational treatment.

And I propose that the therapist/analyst's task in each and every treatment involves a particular focus on the reclamation and growth of the availability of Body Words in both participants. I believe that Body Words experience, in whatever form it takes, provides the singular key to unlocking stubborn repetitions.

Doreen and Me

At this writing, I am shocked to discover myself unable to conjure Doreen's face. And yet I have a sense of certain modes of being that her face gets into, like eyebrows slightly raised, eyelids half-mast along with a sideways glance that marks disdain; or her closed-mouth, tight-lipped so-called smile that tells me *she has had enough of that*! But it's almost as if these looks of hers are happening to *me*! And living behind my face as I do, I remain blind to the contours of Doreen's responses while feeling them intensely.

That said, I do remember exactly what she's wearing on that first day she comes to see me—a moss-green business suit and the simplest, most buttery brown leather pumps you could imagine! *Bruno Magli*, I think to myself, *or what's his name? Blah blah Blahnik ... Manolo Blahnik! My goodness, wow!!*

Doreen married straight out of college to a good man and was already established in her career before she had her first two children, but I have no idea of a husband and family on the day that I first lay eyes on her. Nor am I aware of her desire to bear another child in spite of the gratifications of a prominent position in the business world and two miscarriages as well. I place her in her early thirties. Innocent and tense, and somewhat breathless. My mother would have labeled her "high strung." And, I would add, well heeled.

After standing for a moment in the doorway and briefly checking out my space with her eyes, she gestures a royal greeting with a wave of her right hand as she moves toward the couch, leaving the door open behind her. I close the door and invite her to sit, which she does, perching on the edge of the couch at the end farthest from my chair. Doreen is very tall and slender, the kind of woman who can cross her legs and pretzel one heeled foot around the other ankle and hold it there in the grip of a figure eight. An amazing feat by my lights. Maybe it is my impression of her perfect pose in tension with some unspoken pain that leads me to kind of flop myself down in my chair like a kid to hear her story. *Searing pain*, I think to myself, *yet something thin about it ... disconnected.*

A month ago Doreen's father had died suddenly, alone in the night. In her shock and sorrow Doreen, estranged from her mother and two siblings, feels alone. It seems there is no one to turn to. "People don't want to keep hearing about your troubles," she tosses off, half laughing. "You lose friends that way."

I was, in a softening way, actually able to be in something with Doreen during the first six months of tears that carry us to moments of genuine yearning and sorrow. But once she has reviewed the details of the distance between herself and her sibs—a younger brother and his twin sister, whom she named "the favored ones"—once we took the time together to go over and over what happened, it begins to feel routine. I push a bit with an inquiry about certain feelings. Are they new to her, is there any way they feel familiar? And briefly, I learn about the day in eighth grade when she comes home from school to both her parents sitting in the living room, waiting to break the news of their divorce. But I can't go there. I try.

From where I sit now, perusing my process notes from years ago, I pause to wonder how my inquiry contributed to Doreen's shutting of her door. Was I thoughtless, or clumsy? Nothing like that appears in my notes. But I associate to myself as a little kid, maybe six or seven, having knock-down-drag-outs with my sister. Two years older. She was the quiet one who kept to herself, who often chose to read her book rather than play with me. I am aching for her company. Her inscrutability puts me in a rage. So what is it with Doreen? Is she angry with my knocking on her door, asking her these questions? Am I the only one who wants to play?

She tells me, a slight edge in her voice, how her mother never cried, tells me almost as if she holds me responsible for her revealing that, and how her mother had always been remote from her children. As we review the story about her parents' announcement of divorce for a few more sessions, Doreen gradually recedes, leaving me to sit with the echo of her scent—Lily of the Valley—and odd strings of sentences I could observe from the movement of her lips, like the sound went off, and I am watching a silent movie.

Now I have to wonder about the nature of my attributions to Doreen. It could be she was shy, or reticent. What makes me think she's in a fight with me? My superior older sister shut the glass door on my running after her, shut the door and locked it! Who does she think she is, looking down on my tantrums with such disgust? Bigger and smarter than me. Locking the door so I can't get back at her for putting my doll up on the high shelf I can't reach. I pushed at that door, and my whole arm went through the glass, and I was bleeding all over the place. Then she was the one who got in trouble, not me! And just because I bit her thigh when she was on the ladder putting my doll up on the high shelf.

I am smiling thinking about this. Nonetheless, I am certain that I was angry, but so was Doreen.

Every week she comes to see me directly from work, impeccable in a business suit and stylish pumps, and every week I try to reach her.

"How are you?" She smiles as she comes in to sit down.

I smile back and nod. "Yourself?" I inquire.

"Doing okay," nodding, still smiling, "Okay."

There is silence. Doreen lays in wait. So I smile again. (*Why am I doing that, why do I smile?*)

I take a breath, and I ask, "What does that feel like, Doreen? Can you tell me what it feels like, you're doing okay?"

"It feels good to be here," she asserts, nodding. Smiling. Another empty silence threatens, and I just can't stand it! I want to stomp my feet.

"Last week," I say to her, "you talked about your sister not inviting you and your kids to her daughter's birthday party." (*Why am I falling for this? I wonder, teetering on outrage. What am I doing here??*) "Tell me what happened with that."

"With what?" she answers, abstractly, absorbed in my flowers on the cabinet across from where she sits.

"Your sister, your feelings about that."

"Oh, I just got over it," Doreen sighs. "She is who she is, she's not going to change."

And so the session continues. Once more, I am observing her lips move in a pattern that details her sister's unrecognizing behavior in various situations. *She is not my sister now*, I think to myself, *and she is talking about us*. I fling my feet up on the footstool in front of me. (The footstool that matches my so-called stressless chair! *Right.*)

Doreen goes on with some diatribe about an underling at work, and we are both disappearing. "Helpless" does not quite fit what I am feeling. Tears and outrage, hers and mine, mixed with what? I dig my fingernails into the palm of my hand to stay awake. I wonder which one of us is telling the other that we're done. I am feeling clumsy … ungainly. And I am struck by the sight of my shoes—from the vantage point of my chair—glaringly inappropriate for a therapist at work …

What is this strange business with my shoes, I wonder, as I sit alone writing up my notes. I flag the question in red, which is my promise to return to it at some later opportunity, which if I did, I don't remember.

Now it comes to me from nowhere, a long-forgotten aphorism: "If the shoe fits, wear it." Wow!! Russell (2006a) emphasizes that "The most important source of resistance in the treatment process is the therapist's resistance to what the patient feels" (p. 618).

I experience a flash of guilt and shame. What comes to me is the memory of walking home from school having to face my mother wearing Carley

Stone's shoes. Caught! Borrowing stuff without permission—even among us sisters—was a definite *No-no* in our household. My parents were Hitler refugees, and I went all through grade school during the Second World War. I didn't understand exactly what it was about me that caused the kids to call me "Nazi" or "Jew" (mostly behind my back, but I heard it), but everything about me shouted out my foreignness, including what my mother called my *sensible shoes*. All the other girls are wearing kid's loafers, or saddle shoes, or even Mary Janes on special days while I am stuck in my clunky, brown lace-up, double-toe Oxfords.

One morning (I forget what grade—maybe first or second), I convince Carley that it would be fun to trade shoes, just for the day, which we do. But then it happens that Carley throws up all over her desk, and her mother comes to get her and take her home. I must have been really upset, because it is only in the afternoon in the middle of my walking home that I realize I have to face my mother in Carley's Mary Janes …

And with this long-forgotten memory, another one attaches itself, one that I wrote up some twenty years ago about myself as a youngster on the sidewalk in the dark of a winter night, and it is cold, and I am walking home next to my sister and my mother. A late winter night in January—maybe it is snowing—and suddenly my mother pushes me, pushes both of us forward into the dark. "Run ahead children, *run ahead!*"

My mother was unbelievably private about her person, and it wasn't like her to raise her voice. I hardly ever saw her cry. Now without warning or explanation, she is pushing us away from the comforting presence of her body, shoving us forward in the dark. And then through the darkness I *hear* these intense, guttural-wracking sounds and an incomprehensible splatter. I feel certain that without me near enough to protect her, she is being cut apart and bleeding. I can feel my feet stamping on the cold sidewalk, wetness up through the soles of my shoes. I can hear my own wailing deep inside my head, *Mommy is dying, Mommy is dying!* And then, I remember the comic relief that isn't funny at the time. "Barbara," chides my elder sister, who manages upsets with disdain, "Mother is throwing up."

My mother tells us we are going to have a baby sister. Now the memories of childhood loneliness and feeling left out float in like distant music. I find myself reliving all sorts of childhood scenes that have to do with clumsy efforts to get closer to whatever it was I felt certain my sister had that made our mother love her best—"the favored child," Doreen would say. I think about Doreen. Doreen's shoes and mine. So opposite and yet … Are we like those Scotty-dog magnets with our backs to one another? When all I would have to do is turn around.

Now our deepest yearnings feel familiar.

I realize that the thought of suggesting we had reached the end of our work constituted *my* wish to run away from affective connection. We were both caught in interlocking transferences. I realize that whatever it was that belonged to Doreen, I had turned my back on her. And as I told you at the very outset, I could have lost Doreen before it was her time to go.

If the treatment relationship is to survive, Russell (1994) says, *if the treatment is to take place at all*, patient and therapist will have to *be in it together* and importantly survive together the two major organizing crises that must inevitably, repeatedly ensue if real growth or transformative change is to occur.

The first major crisis consists of the patient's bringing to the therapist/analyst his unquestioning certainty that she will respond to him in the same familiar ways that led him to seek treatment in the first place. The second major crisis comes about with the discovery that the analyst does not match the patient's repetitious transference expectations, a crisis that carries with it the potential opening of an intimate human relational space. But never mind. The patient's sense of self and reality is destabilized, and there is high stress in the consulting room. And beyond all that, the very opening of potential ushers in along with it the grief and pain of how it might have been all along and wasn't.

I didn't have it written in my blue journal, but I imagine that the memories I just described freed me somehow from my repetitions so I could soften and feel more connected to Doreen. If my memory serves me, I believe I made the first move in that direction. Instead of suggesting to her that we'd done our work, we carry on, and over time there is indeed a change in our relating. I wish I had recorded more about it in the blue journal that I keep above my desk. But somehow the feelings between us melt into something else, which I intend to show.

Moving toward the Second Crisis

Russell (1994) explains that repetitions need to be replaced with a relationship for growth to occur. In such a therapeutic relationship, a patient discovers "who the therapist is, *as therapist*," and when that happens, Body Words can be discovered and expressed.

It is precisely that discovery that gives words, gives feeling to all the ways in which this experience was not there before, the ways in which what happened before was different. The technique of therapy [or analysis] consists of the therapist's being able to survive the attempt at coerced identity and to emerge as in fact different. (p. 215)

Let me fast forward to a brief vignette that describes an interaction between us just about two years later. I have deliberately chosen a section in which the precise content of our concerns remains unclear. Elucidating the content would only distract from showing you how Body Words naturally evolve.

"You'd think that I'd *know* better," she said.

"I guess." It came out tentative, noncommittal.

"You'd *think* that I would … " She seemed to be rolling the words around inside her head like so many marbles. "And the truth of it is that I do. But that didn't stop me from doing it."

"No," I agree.

"Am I self-destructive?"

"In this case, I suppose you could call it that … " I shrug. "I don't really know."

"But self-destructive doesn't square with my experience."

In the ensuing silence I think to myself, this is new behavior. I sense that her struggle doesn't have to do with me anymore, that she's no longer caught in the repetitions that caused her to close the door on me. Now there's a chance for her to discover who I am as therapist, as Russell (1994) would say, which constitutes the second crisis of the treatment.

Doreen continues, "It feels to me more like a reaching out than shutting down, or shutting off, or destroying myself." Doreen, who has increased her sessions to three and sometimes four days a week, comes to see me one of those days in her running clothes, and I note that despite her perfect figure, she has the little tummy that mothers end up having no matter how fit they get. I am oddly pleased.

"Funny," she repeats the thought, "more like reaching out. Almost feels like … like a calling."

A picture flashes in my mind. I see my mother, sitting by the door holding onto something above her—as if to a subway strap. Like the subway is jiggling, and she doesn't say a word. I think she is in pain, but she is very quiet. Her eyes are gone. Now I know she was in labor with my youngest sister, who could have come out right there with mother holding onto the strap or whatever it was. She was so *quiet*. It was during the war—not a taxi to be found—and my godmother, hysterically running around on the street calling the police, because nobody would answer the phone. Mrs. Orr would finally come to drive my mother to Lenox Hill. I can't think if she looked back at all, yet I seem to recall her voice, "Don't worry, children," but I can't remember if anyone called anyone to stay with my sisters and me while she was gone.

"A calling?" I say to Doreen, "Like a profession you mean? Or somebody calling?"

"Yeah. Like I have to complete something that was started before I had anything at all to do with it."

I know that Doreen has left her answer ambiguous. I'm used to that, that's the place where I would usually jump in to help. I don't know, but I don't think she does it on purpose. I do know enough by now to know that I won't directly pursue my question at this moment. It feels to me like something is moving somewhere. I want to come along, and I know I cannot. I am intrigued.

"It's happened before, you know it," she adds.

"The calling you?" I ask.

"Yes."

The literal content of Doreen's repetition isn't new to us. We have experienced it many times together in a variety of forms, this business of looking for mother. The new thing here relates to her burgeoning awareness that she is sharing with me some piece of whatever the thing is that is happening now.

For a moment, I can feel myself rail against it. I am tempted to regard her repetition as the same-old same-old even though when push comes to shove, I do know better. I am wanting to go back. Every time this repetition comes around, there's something new to find that we engage in if we feel like it. I am decidedly not feeling like it now. And now I wonder rebelliously if the time has come to name the thing once and for all. Just give it a name and explanation, and then it will go away. Right? *Wrong!*

Whose repetition is this anyway? Is anybody there? The visceral experience we share is not *between* us. It feels different. A pull that doesn't have to do with a tug of war but powerful—compelling! My eyes begin to burn. I notice my throat is dry. "Doreen, what is going on for you? I can't exactly tell what's happening."

What comes to mind is Russell's (2006c) notion that "The expertise in the field consists of the capacity to be aware of, and to effectively repair the interruptions of connectedness that occur by virtue of the therapist's own internal processes" (p. 47). That is, the therapist's resistances. Of course, patients don't necessarily need to know what is going on inside their analyst's mind, but they do need to know that we don't know. What we can try to know, however, again and again, is the part we play in cutting our patient off from what she needs to feel because of some interruption in attachment—of affective connectedness—within ourselves. It's worth repeating, "The most important source of resistance in the treatment process is the therapist's resistance to what the patient feels" (Russell, 2006c, p. 47).

Body Words between patient and clinician, between any two people intimately engaged, move experiencing beyond explanation and meaning, leading to those moments when suddenly something opens up. Body Words create those experiences of movement when sensation/perception has crossed a threshold, and at best, the words—for the first time and only for that time—have captured and created a new integration. Body Words experience comes to life at the point of an ending that potentiates a new beginning.

Body Words evoke a dual process—an intrapsychic dialectic with the potential also to radiate into the intersubjective field and back again, a kind of rising tide in which each successive wave builds on the one that came before. Tide serves well as a metaphor, because there is a kind of draw toward transformation. In Russell's (2006b) terms, when repetitions are *rendered*, we experience the emergence of a new level of affective competence that is the growing edge of owning affect.

Now Doreen is talking about how tired she is, how the two kids and now the baby are such a fulltime job that there is nothing left for her. She needs a little more time before she can return to her "*job*" job. "And with Peter gone all day, he doesn't seem to get it ... although he does ... but ... he's so good with the kids but he doesn't understand and he's so critical of the way I do stuff..." The blood is rising in Doreen's cheeks. "I'm really bummed out that we don't have a village!"

I nod.

Suddenly Doreen says, "*Oh!* I forgot to tell you last time about my dream!"

My stomach flips over. "After the fight with Peter?" I inquire.

"Yes." She shifts her body forward. "You know I'm always having these dreams of me being with the children and, like, not getting some place that we need to get to, or," Doreen laughs, "forgetting to feed the baby!"

"I remember those," I groan. "Horrible."

"Anyway, I had to get to the baby. Brad and Janet were with me." (*I am suddenly confused by the names, Brad and Janet, sibs or kids? In the moment I forget.*) "They were right with me as usual and something kept happening to one of them that prevented me from getting the baby. . . " Doreen stops speaking. And then,

"Here is where I usually wake up. I never get there. But this time I told myself *in the dream, 'no damn it, I'm going to get her.'* And I got her before I woke up. She was there and I got her!" Doreen smiles over this victory.

"Wow, I say. "That is a good dream!"

She agrees.

But it had not occurred to Doreen that the baby might be herself. Nevertheless, this time she seems to accept my suggestion of that possibility.

And I can't tell you how, but I believe that both of us are aware that Doreen is preparing us to talk about the traumas of her early childhood when there is nobody, nobody to hear her calling.

Writing Body Words

Now I would like to return us to the beginning of this narrative, around the time when I first met, and nearly lost, my chance to deepen the work with Doreen. It was just in that time that Body Words came into focus. Here, from my blue journal, is a piece of what I wrote back then.

Within and between self and other, Body Words is my metaphorical term for the experience that leads us to know whether we or the person talking to us is delivering his message in a manner that feels real, or more generally, if the contact we pick up between ourselves and others has a genuine ring to it. By assigning an interactive double name to the phenomenon, I hope to heighten awareness of a dual process involving both the body and the mind without privileging one over the other. Body Words is the corporate version, the communication aspect, the relational edge of the mind/body/brain.

Body is meant to signify the internal corporeal location wherein genuine affects arise and are discretely felt but remain evanescent until or unless words grab hold. *Words*, in this context, serve as a metaphor for affective communication—both verbal and nonverbal—within and between bodies in the larger world. The metaphor bridges affect and cognition. While heartfelt sensations occur in the body, words—a communicable form of expressiveness—provide the containers that permit one's affects to travel around and out.

The circle or process arc of a Body Words experience, in which a body sense is linked to word representation (symbolization, formulation) that becomes communicable to self or other, is always moving. First, a slight interruption of ordinary being makes a bid for attention, a kind of inkling, an itch, a tension in the body that may be ignored, denied, dissociated, or distanced by isolation of affect. But if we choose to turn our attention to that embodied inkling (Gendlin, 1962, 1978 would call it "felt referent"), we become open to discover or have the potential to find words that emerge in our minds—Body Words. This part of the process would be called "carrying forward" in Gendlin's (1978) model of Focusing, or, in Donnel B. Stern's (1997) terms, "formulating experience." The Body Words (gesture or language expressing bodily feelings) can be received and responded to (by analyst or self), and a close observing or listening to the words may induce a further embodied response (for Gendlin, 1978, "referent movement").Thus the circle of Body Words experience may continue as an emergent process that Russell (1994) would call "affective connectedness."

In short, the concept Body Words is what I made of a familiar happenstance in life and therapy. I wrote and rewrote until I reached a kind of settlement that the words I chose came close enough to my experience. Words contain the history of a moment in time as well as provide a context for further transformation.

I confess that when I feel particularly stuck or baffled by a clinical situation, I might ask my patient if she would allow me to write about our work. And that, concretely, is how this chapter actually began, with Doreen's permission and my commitment to finding Body Words within myself that would help me hold the treatment long enough for each of us, from our differentiated roles, to find our way, *to be in* the healing relationship, to give up the safety of aloneness for the safety of affective connectedness (Russell, 1994).

References

Gendlin, E. (1962). *Experiencing and the creation of meaning*. Glencoe, IL: The Free Press of Glencoe.

Gendlin, E. (1964). A theory of personality change. In P. Worchel & D. Byrne (Eds.), *Personality change* (Ch. 4). New York, NY: John Wiley and Sons.

Gendlin, E. (1978). *Focusing.* New York, NY: Random House.

Russell, P. L. (1994). Process with involvement: The interpretation of affect. In L. Lifson (Ed.), *P. Understanding therapeutic action: Psychodynamic The interpretation concepts of cure* In (pp. 201–216). Hillsdale, NJ: The Analytic Press.

Russell, P. L. (2006a). Trauma, repetition, and affect. *Contemporary Psychoanalysis, 42*(4), 601–620. https://doi.org/10.1080/00107530.2006.10747133

Russell, P. L. (2006b). Role of loss in the repetition compulsion. In G. Schamess (Ed.), *Smith college studies in social work, 76*(1/2), 85–98.

Russell, P. L. (2006c). The compulsion to repeat. In G. Schamess (Ed.), *Smith College studies in social work, 76*(1/2), 33–49.

Stern, D. B. (1997). *Unformulated experience: From dissociation to imagination in psychoanalysis.* Hillsdale, NJ: The Analytic Press.

Chapter 16

Coda—Bodies and Embodiment, 1963

The Person of the Analyst

In the final days preparing this book to submit to the publisher and while rummaging through a box of old family papers, I came across an essay I wrote in 1963, nearly a decade before beginning graduate studies in psychology. As I read the forgotten document, it hit me that this brief piece—written in another lifetime when I was Barbara Massar, married to my first husband, and our children were six and four—reflected both the person of the analyst and my earlier experience as an implicated person—rendered no less in body words. So, I have chosen to include this essay, which can be read as an extended reverie.

The Jackson City Jail is full of echoes, and I heard the footsteps of the guard approaching long before he had to tap against the cell window for my attention.

"Barbara Massar!"

"Yes, sir?"

"Come over here so's I can talk to you."

"Sir?"

"You been in here three days. You been tried, you been found guilty, you been sentenced to four months. You been appealed an' Lawyer Hall is downstairs right this minute with your bail. Now I'm not threatenin' you, you understand. I just want to ask you a question."

"Yes?"

"If we arrange to have your bail go through, if we let you get outa here, what will you do?"

"Go home," I answered.

He eyed me testily. "I bet you won't. I bet I'll see you right back in this cell tomorrow, or the next day."

I shook my head.

DOI: 10.4324/9781032666303-26

"Your place is with your husband and your children," he whispered. "That's where you belong."

"I will go home," I told him softly.

And later when the jailer with his strap of heavy iron keys unlocked the door marked "WOMEN WHITE," my first reaction was a surge of joy because the worst was over, and I'd been released at last.

Yet I was wrong. And sometimes when I sit alone with thought too long, it frightens me to find myself regarding jail in Jackson, Mississippi, as less confining than the quaint New England village where I live.

But I should start from the beginning—

I'm twenty-eight. My children—Andrea and David—are six and four. I married young, and until recently it seemed impossible that I could ever separate myself from those on whom I so habitually depended. My husband, Ivan, leaves home all the time. As a magazine photographer, assignments often take him out of town. But even then I'm not alone. There's always Mrs. Carpin, our widowed housekeeper, who's been in the family for years. A hefty, dark, explosive woman, she reminds me of a mother bear—especially the way she guards us with a stern administration of her "loving care."

She and I were watching television on the morning that the news showed the sit-in demonstration in the Jackson, Mississippi, Woolworth store. Lewd and laughing teenagers closed in on the stoic college students at the lunch counter, squirted mustard on their heads, emptied ketchup bottles in their hair. Certainly the sight was no more hideous than the hatred on display in Birmingham or Oxford. But where all previous atrocities set me aflame with righteous indignation, the Jackson filming put me into contact with myself and what was happening like an electrical connection.

Typically, I focused on the stony-faced professor sitting with his students. And suddenly the pride this person evoked was shattered by a blinding sense of shame. Somebody socked him in the eye. All at once I caught myself in the middle of a dreadful act of immorality. They started pouring salt into his bloody wound. What strange conceit inspired me to take so freely of another man's experience? What sort of liberality had I allowed myself whereby I took a stand apart and in the shadows like some "peeping Tom," participating in the agonies and climaxes of other people's living? And in doing that so long, I had developed the audacity to feel their struggle as my own!

A burly expoliceman knocked a Negro[1] to the floor and kicked him in the face—in the face again and again.

"Somebody help!" I gasped.

"Fight back you crazy Negro!" shouted Mrs. Carpin from behind me.

"No, that's wrong, I keep on telling you." Turning to Mrs. Carpin, I discovered that the children had come back into the kitchen and were hanging on her dress enthralled. *"For God's sake get them out of here!"* I yelled.

Swiftly she complied, despite their crying protests, and her movements—like an undercurrent in the din—drew my attention to her silent rage. "I didn't mean to yell," I called out to the yard, "honestly." Mrs. Carpin made no indication that she heard. The news was over. I turned the television off. In an effort to clear my head I sank down at the breakfast table with the fingers of both hands pressed hard against my temples.

So this is how you bring up kids, I thought. First you fill them full of trust, and then you train them in the virtues such as loving and sharing and telling the truth no matter what.

You take them to church and you send them to school and you help them learn their daily pledge and then you're trapped and there is no way out. You're trapped because like "love" and "truth," your country's "liberty and justice" is an all-or-nothing proposition, and if you have to chase the children from the kitchen to protect their innocence, you are preparing for that day when they will fit you in with the rest of the world and never will forget how mother taught white lies.

Mrs. Carpin strode into the kitchen.

"School bus come for Andrea?" I asked.

She nodded. With casual precision, she leaned back on the stove, folded her huge brown arms across that massive chest of hers and waited.

I knew what she was waiting for, to see if I would dare bring up the subject of nonviolence again, to see if I could find among my ready favorites (Jesus, Thoreau, Gandhi, Martin Luther King) some quote explaining why I'd been ashamed to let my children witness the great principle in practice.

I preferred her temper to this new inscrutability against the stove, this mute indifference. She stood there rubbing on her upper arm as if to soothe some burning pain, as if to say "your pretty speeches don't put me to sleep at night, don't make it easier for me to look into my mirror and respect myself. So you take all your holier-than-thou beliefs and put them in a pile and let me know how it stands up against the hell that's going on in Jackson."

That was Wednesday morning, May 29, 1963. I spent the next morning with Alan Gartner, Boston's head of CORE, the afternoon with my children, and the early evening driving into town with Ivan where I kissed him good-bye and boarded the bus for Jackson, Mississippi.

Summer dusk. The bus backed out of the depot groaning through its nose and, with a wheeze of resignation, headed toward the open highway. I squeezed my eyelids shut to minimize the image of my husband heading home alone. Not yet. Not yet. Wait until the dark to cope with the images.

Numbly, I became aware that I had actually made it on the bus without once asking Ivan for permission. This whole business wasn't like me. Not after nine years of such a wifeliness that even when we'd cross the street, I wouldn't pay attention to the traffic, just hang onto his arm, and let him lead me through. By what odd contradiction then, what fear and what desire had mixed up in me that I should suddenly require him to give up my providing for a week or two and every single ounce of his protective instinct! I squeezed my eyelids shut.

Such a sacrifice was just too much to ask of any man. I could not add the burden of permission to it. I could only tell him how I felt I ought to help to deserve the role of mother, citizen, and, in an abstract way, the woman he loved. And we had spoken only briefly—keeping in the silences our common knowledge that if Ivan said, "I cannot let you go to Jackson," I would never mention it again.

But instead he said, "Are you prepared to sit in jail?"

"I don't intend to get in any fistfights, Ivan."

"Then what," he said, "are you planning to bear witness to?"

"There are people in our country," I retorted haughtily, "whose basic civil rights have been denied. Now I'm allowed to say so if I happen to believe it—it's a free country … "

"And if that's the point you want to make," he said, "you can't avoid the jail. Bearing witness is no bargain, Barbara, and unless you're willing to pay full price, I can't afford to finance you."

"All right. I will."

"Then find out about the bail. Speak to somebody who knows what's going on and where you're needed most. After all," he said, "if you want to do some good beyond your own self-satisfaction, you had better find out where the best place is to do it."

It struck me with considerable wonder that, for all my high-flown principles, I'd never tried to contact any of the local action groups. My only membership was in the Unitarian Church whose sermons on "The Preciousness of Every Human Life" and "Man's Responsibility to Man" had taken me no farther than the Sunday Evening Seminars held in the parlor.

"You must really think I'm nuts," I half apologized to Alan Gartner, "and maybe there's a lot more I can do right here instead. I'm ready to contribute any way you say."

He consulted with his New York office and relayed the verdict. This particular weekend, the most important contribution could be made in Jackson.

I didn't understand quite what the contribution was yet couldn't seem to gather up the words to question it. Thursday already, May 30, Memorial Day. "Do you know of many housewives, Alan, who go down and do this sort of thing?"

"I know one."

"Who?"

"You."

"Check with Jackson to make sure," I said, remembering a time when I was young and at a carnival and standing on the roller-coaster line with ropes on either side and people shoving me up forward from behind. A small insistent whim had set itself to motion, gained momentum, caught me in its whirlwind, and had dropped me down and left me at the mercy of a moving bus.

The numbness of my leaving was replaced now by another numbness coming from the sound of speed into a dark unknown and the air conditioning that blasted at my feet (I should have had the sense to bring a coat!) and the exhausting effort to combat regret. Taunted by recall of sleep in my own bed—the whiteness of the sheets, the feel of Ivan's back against my side—I told myself the next stop was New York, and when I got there, all I had to do was turn around.

I walked into the Port Authority Terminal at 2 a.m., a huge and dimly yellow place with the smell of disinfectant rising through the stale remains of vanished crowds. I wondered where to go. According to the timetable, I had to spend an hour in New York. There was something, though, familiar in the atmosphere, a concentrate of long-forgotten nightmares. I hurried toward the restroom, swinging a wide arc around the shouting Negro and the cursing Irishman engaged in drunken warfare. The police had separated them when I came out. They left the Negro sitting on the bench immobile and were dragging the aggressor toward a door and telling him to go on home and sleep it off. I went over to the line of phone booths and considered. Who could I call up at this ungodly hour? I dallied at the newsstand, checked the buses back to Boston, and at last allowed the rolling stairs to take me to the lower platform where the bus to Washington and all points south departed.

The cold grey dawn. Memorial route through Washington. Washington Memorial, Capitol Building, Jefferson Memorial, Lincoln … I saw it as I saw it when my grandmother had taken me after grade-school graduation. A perfect gift, she had decided, for the first in the family born in America. Freedom child—that was me. Richmond.

Richmond to the Carolinas, evening and into Georgia. Strange Land. Why? Ivan and I had come this way before, our children had been born here, we had lived below the Mason Dixon Line for three whole years! But then it was a slightly different South. The lid was on it still, the bubbling ingredients had not boiled over yet, and if we didn't like the scent of south-ern cooking, nobody was forcing us to stay. Certainly it wasn't up to us to change the recipe.

"How long will I have to stay in jail?" I'd said to Alan Gartner at the bus station.

"CORE leaves that decision up to you," he answered. "Jail is a uniquely personal and often dangerous experience. You're completely at the mercy of … "

Union Springs. A hideous accident ahead—a car hung half-way off the mountain road, and, to my utter horror, the bus came to a stop beside it. Three men lay scattered face down in the lush green grass.

"You got help comin'?" called our driver to the people who stood staring by the highway's edge.

"Yes."

And I experienced a strange relief. The pressure that had steadily increased since I left Boston lifted. I felt like I had just come out of major surgery.

"Sure there's nothin' I can do?" the driver called.

"Sure."

And we moved onward through the morning sunshine toward Montgomery, Meridian, and Jackson, Mississippi.

Now the bus made frequent stops along the countryside to pick up local passengers—plantation workers, I supposed. Sitting in the front seat watch-ing them come on—eyes averted and self-contained, I wondered if my pres-ence made the slightest bit of difference to them. No. These were strangers whom I'd never meet. But maybe on this lonely trip below the many layers of my own convention there might be something left of me to get in touch with. And maybe that would be some common thing that touched these people too, but they were not my first concern. I'd seen the nature of my first concern. I had, at least, pulled out that weed of fear that had been choking me so long. I'd grabbed hold of it when I left Boston, and soon after that I tried to let it go again because I sensed that at the very root *I did not want to die!* and this seemed much too corny to take stock of. But resistance only loosened the protective soil that kept the fear embedded. I could not return it to the depths from where it sprung. I could only yank it up through consciousness and struggle with the horror of its possibility.

And then for the first time ever, I had witnessed death strewn in three persons by the highway. I'd seen lush green grass beneath the faceless dead and realized what my fear had been attached to. All I really wanted was a chance to live! "Oh, please," I pleaded silently, "I want to come to life before I die. I'm almost there. Just let me get there in the open once and try. I'm not asking for eternity, but just a little bit of living worth my while."

We crossed the Jackson city line. Whatever sort of jail they had, I knew it would be roomier than where I'd been. I was ready to take my chances now, glad for the opportunity before it was too late.

I took a taxi to the Masonic Hall where the civil rights groups met. I walked into the hall and there—toward the back—stood forty Negro children in parade formation. Attracted by their neat white shirtwaists, I moved closer. They were holding small American flags, and they were singing "We shall overcome, We shall overcome," which made it radiantly clear that what I'd seen and pleaded for aboard the bus was nothing new to them. I never heard such singing, never saw a bunch of kids so totally unhampered by their puberty, so unbewildered, and so filled with purpose. They embodied all I ever read about The Spirit of '76 and showed me that my recent revelation was, in fact, a revolution old as human history. "The truth will make us free," they sang, and the wisdom of it shone like captured sunlight in the dark smooth satin of their foreheads. Forty children ready to march. I followed them out into the blazing street, these forty unarmed children, and I listened to the giant roar close in on them—enough blue-helmeted policemen for a presidential motorcade! Big policemen swinging billy clubs, white citizens with heavy guns strapped to their heavy hips—all mobilized to snatch up children for the crime of a flag and a song and a wish to walk free.

"Where," I whispered to the Negro man beside me, "is the jail?"

"They rigged a special one for children on the Fairgrounds. The stinking exhibition buildings. They took the animals away so there'd be room enough to push the children in. And then they strung it all around with hog-wire."

The kids were singing still inside the paddy wagons—"We are not afraid." But soon the paddy wagons drove away, and there was nothing left except the sunset and the dust. The few adults, like me, who hadn't been arrested, moved as a receding tide along the silent street—and back into the hall.

Reverend Edwin King, his tall frame sagging slightly, leaned against the water fountain talking to his wife. "Well, at least they didn't throw them in the garbage trucks this time. The kids were really frightened by the garbage trucks."

A gentle sigh from Mrs. King.

"I'm ready to participate," I said.

"You've only just arrived!"

How odd that I should have forgotten that. "Listen, if those kids can do it."

"The best thing you can do," said Ed, "is stay around awhile. Talk to as many people as you can. Get to know them. Tell them where you come from, who you are, and why you've come. Ask them all the questions that you want."

Really odd. I felt like I had been in Jackson half a lifetime, like I'd always known the Kings. Ed was Chaplain at Tougaloo, an integrated college just outside the city, and Jeannette was everything that made him possible. The two were white-born Mississippians ("Southern traitors") whose dedication to the freedom movement kept them in a constant state of danger.

"You must be tired from your trip," Jeannette said sympathetically, "Come on, we're going to take you home."

Home, for the next few days, was with the Kings. We commuted back and forth between the college and the hall—police cars tailing everywhere we went. And I suppose it was the constant danger and the common cause that heightened the importance of each tiny moment and welded brief acquaintance into friendship.

I slept in a room with the Salter baby. John and Eldrie brought her over every night because whoever shot into their house had sent his bullet through the nursery window. And as I realized that a freedom song would someday weave around the pale and stony-faced Professor Salter, I could understand his inaccessibility. His pain was too intense for anyone to bear, and out of courtesy to others, he would fold it back into himself. His smile, with just his lips, was like the sealing of an envelope.

It surprised me that Negroes were more open with emotion. I observed the children who had been through jail train younger children in nonviolence: "We got to show them who is beast. The switchblade never showed nobody nothin'." I spoke with Negro mothers, and I asked a lot of questions and began to see into the vastness between "child" and "innocence."

"But when," asked a little boy who watched his friend get thrown into the paddy wagon, "are the Americans coming? When are the Americans coming?"

"And when," I said to Medgar Evers, "will you let me do something!"

"You have already ... just by being here." The warmth and the incredible compassion gathered in his face to tell me that I didn't have to go as far as jail to offer me my ticket home. "Your children must be missing you," he hinted.

"So must yours," I hinted back. "You've been working day and night, but I guess it's all a part of our responsibility to them." "You've come a long, long ways," he smiled, "and I appreciate—"

"Your kids and my kids are going to grow up in the same world, Medgar, and it's getting smaller every day. There's no more room for 'yours' and 'mine' anymore. Our kids are going to have to share whatever world we make for them, and you've been working very hard so please let me do some little thing."

A flash of suffering crossed his face. He sighed. "All right then. Speak at the rally tonight, and we'll let you go out tomorrow."

The thought of speaking to a crowd of people who had been through hell and back embarrassed me. But when I walked across the platform to the lectern and the people rose and rocked me with the ocean-tide of their applause, I understood the message that I carried. "Tell them where you come from, who you are." Well, I'd come out of Massachusetts, and I'd been through Barbara Massar so that these were details now that didn't matter. What mattered was I could be counted as a woman from America who had cared enough to come.

The temperature climbed up the next day to ninety-nine degrees. Shortly before noon, three Negroes and myself walked from the hall to Ed King's car. Mr. Butler took the flag; the rest of us had placards. Florina's said,

"The truth shall not be jailed;" Mrs. Catching's, whose girl had just been beaten in the concentration camp, carried a sign that said, "Do unto our children as you would do unto yours;" and my sign expressed the belief that "When children suffer, all Americans suffer."

"The City Hall," Ed told me as we left the curb, "is set back over a hundred feet from the sidewalk so don't let them convince you you're inciting the emotions of a crowd. There won't be a crowd—not with the policemen and the paddy wagons and photographers."

Something in my chest began to swell and stiffen. I figured maybe I might stall off rigor mortis if I sang. And the others must have thought it was a good idea because they joined in right away. "We shall overcome, we shall overcome ... " All of us together in one voice. And when we got to "We are not afraid," it didn't seem so bad to feel afraid, and what we really meant was we were not afraid to be afraid. "Deep in my heart, I do believe." Clearly, just as long as we kept singing, we could overcome.

"Okay now," Ed instructed, "Mr. Butler, put the flag inside your shirt. You ladies keep your placards rolled until you reach the steps. God bless you."

"The Lord is on our side," we sang quietly to help each other towards the steps.

I had not considered "God" or "Lord" as part of this at all. And as I placed the placard string around my neck, my only thought was to maintain that level that the singing had achieved, to keep my lips in motion. "Our Father," as long as we were on the subject, "which art in heaven..." The sun beat down like lead pipe on my head. "Give us this day ... " I wondered if I'd faint, "and forgive us our trespasses." That is when the thing came over me—the unexpected blessing. I could feel the shape and form of it come up into my mouth "as we forgive those who trespass against us."

"I'm goin' to ask you to move on," said Captain Ray. He had to say it in a microphone to make himself be heard, to say it in the company of a bunch of big policemen with blue helmets, leather belts, and guns.

God, I thought, there ought to be a simpler way than forcing these policemen out into the sun with all that heavy armor on.

"You're blockin' the entrance to City Hall," crowed Captain Ray, "move on."

The City Hall is six miles long, I thought, and we are praying nowhere near the doors. I came here to bear witness, not to make a public fool of you. I don't want to do it. Can't you see you're doing it to yourself? Can't you see!

"I'm goin' to ask you one more time ... move on."

"but deliver us from evil ... "

"All right. You're under arrest."

I'm sorry, Captain Ray. I *really* am.

The Jackson City jail is full of echoes, and the hollow clang of cell doors closing freedom in. The iron cot, the urine stench imbedded in the mattress, the cockroaches, the tin cup, and the filthy toilet open to the jailer's view must be expected and withstood in any prison. And none of these can take away the dignity of right. And there is something to be said for Jackson's jail. When the Negro prison trustee—driven to my window by misguided masters or misguided sex—could see I hadn't come so far for a relationship with him, he let me be. Policemen and detectives spoke with me, at least, gave me the opportunity to overcome hostility and ignorance (the prisoner in WOMAN WHITE was not a Communist, no fanatic; some people believed in liberty and justice just because they thought that it was right). At least I was permitted in the Jackson jail to *meet the challenges!*

And that is not exactly how it is at home. I have been at home three months, and still my three short days in prison make some people feel uncomfortable. And there are attitudes around me that I find more difficult to deal with since they're hidden and unspoken. The Northern "Liberal But" has found excuses for the fear the Southern Bigot has admitted, and the "Liberal Liberal" (that was me!) does not really wish to face the fear at all.

"But Negroes ought to concentrate on their own improvement first," says Liberal But who calls a spade a spade and the kettle black. "But they're biting off the very hand that feeds them!" he exclaims—rejecting peaceful demonstrations that, in fact, comprise his only stay of execution.

And throughout all this the Liberal Liberal remains aloof. I know one who despises agitation—considers it degrading and, if he must say so, uncouth.

"Barbara, you have got to," he will smile a smile identical to Ross Barnett's, "give these people *time!*"

"Time and tide," I try to tell him, but he's up to his ears and cannot hear me anymore.

And it's a shame since I would like to tell him that the time is not for me to give or take away, that the evening is already spread against the sky, the moment at its crisis, and the overwhelming question "Do I Dare" will soon be answered one way or another.

Note

1 In these early days of the Civil Rights Movement, the word *Negro* was the preferred term chosen by the African-American community to describe themselves.

Final Reverie

There Must Not

There must not have been too much going on in the world on the day that I got arrested, because a picture of me being hauled off—Gandhi style— appeared on the front page of the *New York Herald Tribune* and the *Boston Globe*.

Now I no longer remember who told me about the scene with my daughter, Andrea, when I was gone. Was it the kindergarten student teacher, maybe, or a parent observing the class?

Or wouldn't it be a good thing if the teacher herself took Andrea's response to heart and therefore let me in on the conversation that occurred between them in front of the whole class? Here it is.

Teacher: Andrea, where is your mother?
Andrea: In Mississippi.
Teacher: Where in Mississippi?
Andrea: Jackson.
Teacher: Where in Jackson?
Andrea: In the jail.
Teacher: What is your mother doing in jail??
Andrea: (shrugging) Oh, she's gone to find freedom for all of us children.

DOI: 10.4324/9781032666303-27

Index

Miloscz, C.
  "Incantation" (poem) 74
Mitchell, S. 4, 28n1, 57, 64, 70, 80n5, 82,
  94, 145n3
  destructive aggression 162
  intersubjectivity 4–5
  love and hate in the analytic
    relationship 57, 64, 75, 78, 136,
    156–157, 168n4
  role responsibilities of analyst and
    patient 55, 57
  versions of self 158
Modell, A. 19
"Morning Poem" 62
Morrison, A.
  self-disclosure 16
mutative agent 86–87

nonanalytic third 5, 56–57, 65, 69,
  80n4, 84–87
  food as 85–86
  poetry as 5, 77, 79, 110
  September 11, 2001 as 70–74, 77
  and soulful metaphor 5, 87–88

Oates, J. C.
  on power and the Deadly Sins 137
Ogden, T. H. 186–187
  interpretive action 94
old age 221–223, 225–226
  as life's last developmental epoch 225
Oliver, M.
  "Morning Poem" 62
  "The Summer Day" (poem) 228
  "Wild Geese" (poem) 4–5, 65–67, 77
Orfanos, S. 79n1
outrageous interpretation 4–6, 89, 91,
  93–97, 103, 114, 115
outrageous intervention 93, 95, 115

personifications
  old-me 9, 225–226, 229n4
  see also Sullivan, H. S.
Pizer, S. 6, 19, 36, 45, 79n1, 110, 158
  black holes 110, 118
    as relational metaphor for the
    unconscious 113
  Donald (clinical example) 15
  nonanalytic third 80n4
  the nonnegotiable 114, 115
    nonnegotiable stance of a traumatized
    patient 137–138
  shock of recognition 133, 137

poetry 5, 74, 76–77
  in clinical practice 56, 61–67, 74, 79
  as nonanalytic third 56–57, 77, 79, 110
Poland, W. 121
psyche and social
  role of Body Words in 10

Rapaport, D. A. 83
relational (k)not see (k)nots
Renik, O. 17, 21, 26, 28n1
  analyst's personality revealed 28n3
  enactment 14
repetition compulsion 7, 9–10, 33, 34,
  150–151, 153, 164–166, 213
  as black hole 114
  and Body Words 235
  development of 235
resistance 9, 14, 23–25, 138, 151, 166, 238,
  243, 253
Rothko, M. 83, 84
Russell, P. L. 9, 114, 151–152, 157, 164,
  167, 240–241
  affective-cognitive structure 42
  affective competence 33, 243
  affective connectedness 2, 243, 245
  analytic intimacy 156
  containment 33–34, 42, 52
  crisis of attachment 34
  crunch 4, 33–35, 38–40, 110, 111
    affectively laden exchange of
    enactments 33–34
    necessity of 34
    rendering of the repetition 34
  descriptive and prescriptive rules
    209–210, 215–216
  dissociation 151
  essential paradoxes 33
  involvement/noninvolvement 35, 41,
    111, 112, 211
  "The Negotiation of Affect" 210–211
  organizing crises in treatment 240–241
  owning affects and negotiating affects as
    developmental structures 168n5
  owning feelings 235
  paradoxes 40
  process with involvement 41, 53
  repairing interruptions of
    connectedness 243
  repetition and containment 33, 52
  repetition compulsion 33, 34, 151,
    164–166, 213, 235
  resistance of therapist in treatment
    process 9, 238, 243

structure as passage of process with
involvement 53, 211
therapy and affect 39–40

Sam (clinical example) 57–79, 88, 116
firewall 77
poetry 61–66, 74–75
Schore, A. N. 199
self-disclosure 3–4, 6, 13–14, 28n1, 96,
110, 121, 123–124, 129
countertransference disclosure 19–22,
25, 27
deliberate 14, 15, 18, 25–27
inadvertent 14, 15, 19–25, 94, 96
inescapable 14–19
see also Aron, L.; Greenberg, J.
self-system 9, 223, 225
see also Sullivan, H. S.
September 11, 2001 70–74, 77
sexual abuse in analysis 8, 135–137,
207–208, 212–213
Shapiro, F. 191n3
Eye Movement Desensitization and
Reprocessing (EMDR) 188
Silberger, J. 137–139, 146n4
Simon, B. (clinical example) 43–44, 46–53
Solomon, D. 89
Stern, D. B. 2, 4, 57, 69, 70, 73, 79n1, 151,
168, 224, 234
courting surprise 61, 65
enactment 87, 94
formulating experience 2, 245
fusion of horizons 74
interpersonalization of
dissociation 108n2
mutative agent 86–87
nonanalytic third 84–87
on Pizer, B. writing style 5, 81–88
poetry 82, 84–85, 88
relational freedom 4
soulful metaphors 5, 87–88
unbidden word, gesture, or phrase 2, 234
unformulated unconscious 114
Stern, D. N. 109n4
Stern, D. N., Sander, L., Nahum, J.,
Harrison, A., Bruschweiler-Stern, N., &
Tronick, E. 86
Strachey, J. 114

Sullivan, H. S.
interpersonal theory 223
personifications: good-me, bad-me,
not-me 9, 223–224, 229n3
self-system 9, 223, 225
seven developmental stages 224
"The Summer Day" (poem) 228

Dr. T. (clinical example) 22–25
Tansey, M. J. 28n1
training 53n2, 84, 138–139, 206, 209
more needed about affects 212–213
transference 7, 19, 22, 28n4, 140, 157, 164,
201n2, 206, 209, 240
transference/not-transference and not-
transference/transference 19
trauma
metabolizing rather than getting over 216
nightmares moving in slow motion
208, 215
transgenerational transmission 217
treatment process 9, 35, 42, 69, 76, 86, 94,
117, 123–124, 151–152, 158, 163, 175,
178, 206–207, 234, 238, 243
resonant theory 177–178
technique 4, 13–14, 34, 35, 41, 45, 53n2,
56, 95, 121, 124, 209
theory 174–175, 177–178, 183–184

unbidden word, gesture, or phrase 2, 234

Weakland, J. H. 36
double bind 4, 24
"Wild Geese" (poem) 4–5, 65–67, 77
Winnicott, D. W. 21, 26, 52, 94, 178,
186, 187
aggression as intrinsic to maturational
processes 150
"alone in the presence of another/
someone" 178, 186, 187
holding environment 215
writing 5, 9, 81–84, 113, 165, 233, 244
Wu, Y. J. & Thierry, G. 167
bilingual mind and native language
translation 151, 165–166
cognitive unlinking 151
emotion-cognition interactions 165–166

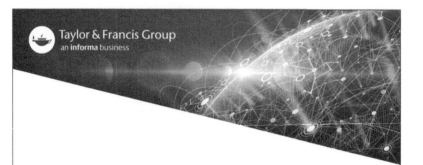

For Product Safety Concerns and Information please contact our
EU representative GPSR@taylorandfrancis.com Taylor & Francis
Verlag GmbH, Kaufingerstraße 24, 80331 München, Germany